THE
BREAST HEALTH
COOKBOOK

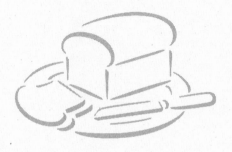

THE
BREAST HEALTH
COOKBOOK

FAST AND SIMPLE RECIPES TO REDUCE
THE RISK OF CANCER

BY ROBERT ARNOT, M.D.

Recipes and Menus by

BARBARA SULLIVAN, PH.D., and RITA MITCHELL, R.D.

LITTLE, BROWN AND COMPANY
Boston   New York   London

First Edition

For information on Time Warner
Trade Publishing's online publishing program,
visit www.ipublish.com.

Library of Congress Cataloging-in-Publication Data

Arnot, Bob.
The breast health cookbook: fast and simple recipes
to reduce the risk of cancer /
by Robert Arnot.
p. cm.
Includes index.
ISBN 0-316-05133-0
1. Breast — Cancer — Diet therapy — Recipes. 2. Breast — Cancer — Prevention.
I. Title.

RC280.B8 A757 2001
616.99'449052 — dc21
00-046942

10 9 8 7 6 5 4 3 2 1

Q-FF

Printed in the United States of America

Book design by Jo Anne Metsch

CONTENTS

Introduction   3

PART I   7

How Foods May Help Protect You from Breast Cancer   9
The Menu Plans   24

PART II ▪ RECIPES   45

Breakfast   47
Soups and Stews   88
Sandwiches   111
Main Courses   120
Main-Dish Salads   166
Side Dishes—Grains and Legumes   178
Side Dishes—Vegetables   192
Side Salads   200
Desserts   221

Index   253

THE
BREAST HEALTH
COOKBOOK

INTRODUCTION

My wife, Courtney, laid down the challenge when she asked a simple question: How do I protect myself from breast cancer? She was young and afraid. Her mother had contracted breast cancer at a strikingly youthful age and Courtney feared for her own health and well-being. After a long and fascinating search, I came back to her with a treasure trove of foods that had powerful effects on the female breast. I laid out the arguments and explained to her how women in the Far East have 90 percent less breast cancer than American women. I explained how scientists believed that foods were what protected these women. I explained in great scientific detail how individual foods uniquely affect the actual biochemistry and even the structure of the very breast duct cells where cancer arises.

To my great surprise, one day after finishing the final manuscript of *The Breast Cancer Prevention Diet*, I found her in the kitchen eating a Philadelphia cheese steak accompanied by fat-soaked spinach pastries and polished off with a pint of high-sugar, low-fat chocolate ice cream. My face fell in dismay. I instinctively reached for the refrigerator and pulled out a burger made of soy. Have this, I offered. No way! she said. As I pulled out one food after another — edamame, soy milk, tofu, miso — my spirits sank. No! No! No! she said. I'd gone to great effort to create a personal program for her, but she wouldn't touch it. Why? I asked in bewilderment. The answer was simple. "Your foods don't taste good," she said. I tried to persuade her that she'd be doing herself so much good that it was worth forgoing great taste. I should have known better; I'd heard it before from food scientists. They used the same word over and over again. Ask for the three most important criteria in designing meals and they will tell you: Taste, taste, taste.

So I set out on a second journey, a journey to create meals with spectacular taste, while still incorporating every last element of a healthy-breast eating plan — meals my wife, my children, and our friends would eat. Pharmacists have long formulated medications by adding many different ingredients. I wanted to formulate the perfect meal that would contain all the right foods in just the right proportions to reduce the risk of breast cancer.

That led me to two remarkable women, Barbara Sutherland, Ph.D., and Rita Mitchell, R.D. Both are first-rate, innovative nutritionists, curious scientists, and great chefs. Both work at the University of California at Berkeley. I asked them to help me create meals that could help prevent breast cancer. They jumped at the chance. They saw this book as the fruition of their lifetime quest to combine the art of cooking with the science of nutrition to prevent disease and promote health.

It came as somewhat of a surprise that Rita's and Barbara's first criterion was the same as my wife's. Their recipes had to taste great. Their "taste" judges were tough: family, friends, and neighbors. But Barbara and Rita were first hard on themselves. Until Rita saw a smile on Barbara's face and heard her exclaim, "It's a knockout!" a recipe did not reach their hard-nosed judges. My first bite of their first recipe hit me square between the eyes. WOW! I thought to myself, that tastes just about as good as any meal could. There were great tastes, subtle tastes, sparkling tastes, all surprising and delighting the palate. Sometimes they got lucky and had a great-tasting dish the first time. Other times they went back to the drawing board again and again looking for inventive ways to make the recipes work and work well with the foods necessary for the plan. It took several attempts — adjusting ingredients or preparation methods — before they got it right. Their philosophy was to develop recipes that tasted great, used fresh ingredients whenever possible, and were quick and easy to prepare

Rita and Barbara succeeded in spades. I now cook these meals myself, easily and quickly. The lure for me and for our family is that the dishes taste so great that they're well worth the small amount of effort it takes to prepare them instead of making a mad dash for the microwave (or the phone to order takeout).

We also learned an important lesson. As our lives have become increasingly frantic, our schedules more jumbled and our days packed with activities, we tend to overlook the importance of food. In this hectic lifestyle, we often grab food on the run or buy fast food to eat in our cars on those vast parking lots known as freeways. Many of us have lost sight of the significance of mealtimes. In addition to providing food and nourishment, mealtimes should be an opportunity to relax and enjoy life. You have to eat; you may as well take the time to select and prepare disease-fighting foods and also take the time to enjoy them! Earlier this year I traveled to Paris for *Dateline NBC*, to interview Professor Claude Fischler, a sociologist who studies eating behaviors. He explained how Americans not only eat badly but are also so conflicted and stressed by their poor food choices that they make an already unhealthy experience even more harmful and emotionally draining. He taught me the tremendous importance of meals as a celebration of life. At the elegant Guy Savoy restaurant in Paris, he showed me how a wonderful meal, great company, and stimulating conversation could strip away stress and create a style of life that gives us more joy and pleasure each day.

In our rushed society, we often view eating as refueling, a pit stop. While we forage for burgers, sodas, muffins, bagels, even candy bars, we miss the centerpiece of good eating — great meals. The recipes in this book can be put together quickly and easily, so you don't have to rely on the local fast-food joints or convenience stores. These are meals around which you can build a great social occasion. In many cases, you can prepare part of the recipe ahead of time, making last-minute cooking a breeze. Eating is an essential part of family and social life, and it can still delight the palate while perhaps saving your life.

Putting yourself on a healthy eating plan doesn't mean limiting your choices; it means expanding them. It doesn't mean barring yourself from exploration. You'll find the foods here offer a great adventure, teaching you about cultures with fabulous culinary traditions and marvelously healthy foods. There are three separate cuisines in the book, each a magnificent series of food adventures: Asian, New American, and Mediterranean. It's your choice: mix and match recipes you like from all three if you have a low risk of breast cancer. For a more intensive regime, you'll first want to consider the Asian recipes.

This book is divided into two parts. Part I begins with a chapter on the science behind the recipes. You'll then find a full description of the Asian, New American, and Mediterranean menus, and a complete set of meal plans. Part II presents the recipes. For your convenience, they are listed in the following categories: breakfast; soups and stews; sandwiches; main courses; main-dish salads; side dishes — grains and legumes; side dishes — vegetables; side salads; and desserts. Within each of those sections you'll find all the Asian recipes together, all the New American together, and all the Mediterranean together.

MEN TOO

One big concern for women who have a family may be, Gee, this food is great and healthy for me, but what about the rest of my family? How can I sell them on a healthy-breast eating plan, especially my husband? There's good reason husbands and wives should share this same healthy eating plan. Why? Ironically, husbands and wives may have a shared cancer risk. Men married to women with breast cancer have a higher risk of prostate cancer. Women married to men with a higher risk of prostate cancer have a higher risk of breast cancer. This correlation between two unrelated individuals underscores the significance of healthy eating (and lifestyle) in the prevention of breast cancer. And brothers and sisters may also share a risk of cancer. Should you have a family history of either cancer and share the BRCA1 gene for breast cancer, the men in your family have a higher risk of prostate cancer. Fortunately, virtually every dietary measure taken to prevent breast cancer is also a vital part of a program to protect the men in the family from prostate cancer. There are some minor modifications to the recipes in this book that target the prostate even more specifically. Those are noted at the end of certain recipes.

(These prostate cancer modifications have been provided at the bottom so that they will be least distracting if men are not included in the household cooking plans.)

An eating plan to protect a man from prostate cancer is more stringent than a healthy-breast eating plan. I myself am on a healthy-breast eating plan. As a man, I've opted for the lowest-fat recipes — found in the Asian sections — because animal fat is the most important food risk for prostate cancer. For women, total fat is not a known risk, so women may want to enjoy the Mediterranean and New American recipes as well. Our whole family eats these meals as a great way to stay trim and energetic while helping to prevent not only cancer but also heart disease, diabetes, and obesity. The study of diet and breast cancer is a young one. Conclusive research is many years from completion. Still, the recipes and menu plans in this book embody a robust diet for your overall well-being.

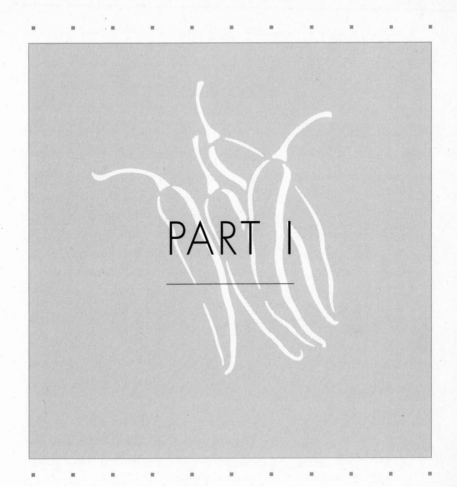

PART I

HOW FOODS MAY HELP PROTECT
YOU FROM BREAST CANCER

I have long believed that foods are the most powerful preventive medicines. Now, sure, no single food is as powerful as a drug, but the elegance of using foods to fight breast cancer is that each class of foods acts in a unique way, quite different from another. By using the different kinds of foods found in this book, you are changing the environment in and around the breast duct cell, where cancer arises, and protecting it. Many researchers believe that the foods women in the Far East eat are the reason they have up to 90 percent less breast cancer than women in America. While some of the foods exert a modest effect independently, together they may have a synergistic effect that gives you a very powerful weapon to use in your own war against cancer. Scientists at the prestigious Cambridge University estimate that as many as 80 percent of breast cancer cases might be prevented with the right eating plan. We won't know the actual benefit until a good deal more research is completed. That's why these recipes are all-inclusive, containing every important food that could protect you against breast cancer.

You might say, Well, gee, if these foods all act in different ways, how do I know how much of each to eat? That's the true genius that Rita and Barbara have brought to this book. Just as pharmacists make up unique formulations to treat illness, each containing several different substances, so, too, recipes are a formulation of foods that combine just the right amounts of all the proper ingredients. By spending hundreds of hours sweating over a stove, Barbara and Rita have created menu plans to meet my specifications.

Let's take a look at the scientific rationale behind the foods that are the basic building blocks of the recipes in this book. For a more detailed discussion of the science, consult my books *The Breast Cancer Prevention Diet* and, for men, *The Prostate Cancer Protection Plan*. You should discuss all your breast cancer early-detection and prevention plans with your physician to customize a program that is best for you based on the very latest scientific data.

SOY

Boy, do I love soy. No kidding! If there is one superfood you'd take with you to a desert island, it's soy. From lowering cholesterol and stabilizing blood sugar to curbing your appetite and improving brain energy, soy does it all. Soy also comes in mouthwatering foods from snap fresh edamame to creamy smooth tofu. Soybeans, a member of the legume family, are native to China and have been farmed there for more than five thousand years. In the United States they have been an important crop for nearly two hundred years. Since soy is one of the highest-quality proteins in nature, consider using soy for most of your protein intake.

BREAST BENEFITS OF SOY

Most researchers believe that estrogen is the key fuel that causes breast cancers to grow. Estrogens may act by increasing cell division and growth. If there is a cancer present, estrogen could facilitate faster growth of the tumor. Evidence shows that women with a greater exposure to estrogen do have a higher risk of breast cancer. For instance, women with an early menarche or late menopause have a higher risk because of the longer lifetime exposure. Their bodies are producing estrogen in peak amounts for more years than those of women with a late menarche or early menopause. Some women produce larger quantities of estrogen, as measured in blood tests, from early in their adult life. They too have a higher risk for developing cancer later in life. One prominent theory holds that soy may help to blunt the estrogen effect. In practice, three studies have observed that women with higher soy consumption run a reduced risk of premenopausal breast cancer. More studies are under way.

The menu plans in this book are high in soy protein, containing on average 35 grams of soy protein per day — approximately 19 grams

Protein Content of Soy Foods Used

mature (dry) soybeans, cooked	½ cup	14 grams
baked tofu	2 ounces	12 grams
fresh green soybeans	½ cup	11 grams
soy tempeh	2 ounces	11 grams
firm tofu	2 ounces	9 grams
soy protein powder	1 tablespoon	8 grams
nonfat soy milk	1 cup	6 grams
silken tofu	2 ounces	3 grams
soy flour	1 tablespoon	3 grams
miso	1 tablespoon	2 grams
tamari soy sauce	1 teaspoon	1 gram

Source: U.S. Department of Agriculture, Agricultural Research Service, 1999. USDA Nutrient Database for Standard Reference, release 13.

come from the meals and an additional 16 grams from a daily soy shake. Following are the soy products used in this book. The table above lists the protein content of common measures of these soy products. Look in the index for recipes using these specific soy products.

SOY CAUTION

One key active component in soy is genistein. This is a weak estrogen. In women with high estrogen production, it may displace powerful estrogens from the estrogen receptors on breast cells, potentially decreasing risk. In women with very little estrogen, genistein may exert its effect as an estrogen. This certainly happens in the test tube, where it may cause existing breast cancer cells to grow. For this reason there are two words of caution. First, don't use any soy product that is "spiked" with genistein or other isoflavones in the soy-shake recipes you'll find in this book. Second, although the overwhelming evidence points to great health benefits for soy in hundreds of millions of women around the world, be sure to consult with your doctor before embarking on a program of regular daily soy ingestion. Be certain it's right for you. In particular, if you are a postmenopausal breast cancer survivor, your doctor may have some reservations. As with any pregnancy, be certain to check with your OB/GYN about soy, fish oils, and any other supplements or medications you may consider taking. If your doctor counsels you against taking soy supplements, you may want to replace soy in the shakes in this book with skim milk.

Fresh Green Soybeans

Until recently, fresh green soybeans could be found only in Asian markets and specialty food stores. Now they are becoming increasingly available in grocery stores throughout the country. Green soybeans are available frozen year-round. However, it's hard to beat fresh soybeans popped right out of the pod for a summertime treat.

Green soybeans are harvested just before they mature and are not left on the bush to dry. Usually soybeans sold in the pods are called fresh soybeans and have been precooked if they are sold in packages. The Japanese term for fresh soybeans in the pods is *edamame*. Refrigerate fresh green soybeans if you plan to use them within a couple of days, or freeze them for longer storage.

If you buy fresh soybeans (not packaged), there are two ways to cook them, depending on how you plan to serve them. For a snack, put the whole pods into lightly salted boiling water for ten minutes. Drain and rinse under cold water. Eat the beans straight from the pod. For use as a vegetable or in mixed dishes, remove the beans from the pods first, then cook the beans in boiling water for about ten minutes.

Mature (Dry) Soybeans

When soybeans are allowed to mature on the bush, they ripen into a hard, dry bean that is light tan or yellow in color. Dried soybeans are commonly available in stores where grains and legumes are sold in bulk. See page 181 for a basic recipe for cooking soybeans. They are easy to cook, and you can prepare them in quantities to have on hand for use in the recipes in this book, as they keep well in the refrigerator for several days.

Cooked mature soybeans are often available canned. They are available in most health food stores and are becoming available in most large grocery chains.

Prepared Black Soybeans

We discovered small cans of prepared black soybeans from Japan in a store with an international foods section. The unique flavor of these beans inspired us to develop several recipes using them. These canned beans had been prepared with water chestnuts and tangles (seaweed), which we removed. For some of the recipes, we rinsed the beans briefly under water. Searching for these beans is well worth the effort.

Tofu

Tofu, also known as soybean curd, is made by first extracting the liquid from soaked crushed soybeans, then making the curd. When prepared with calcium salts (check the label to see if calcium is used), tofu will also contribute to the daily calcium intake.

Fresh tofu is available in different consistencies: extra-firm, firm, medium, and soft, plus silken. The firmer the tofu, the more soy protein it has per serving. Because of this, we have used extra-firm tofu whenever possible. Tofu has a mild taste and easily picks up the flavors of ingredients it is cooked with, making it especially good for use in a stir-fry or curry. Silken tofu is a creamy, custardlike form of tofu and is often used in recipes that call for blending the tofu with other ingredients.

Fresh tofu is available in bulk in Asian markets. In most grocery stores, it is sold in sealed water-filled tubs or aseptic brick packages. Look for it in the refrigerated produce section and store it in the refrigerator at home. If you have leftover tofu, rinse it and cover with fresh water. Change the water daily and use it within a week.

Recently, a variety of flavors of baked tofu, such as savory, teriyaki, and smoked, have come onto the market. Because it has been baked, it has a lower water content and contains more soy protein per serving than fresh tofu.

Soy Tempeh

Tempeh is made from whole cooked soybeans that are fermented, crushed, and formed into cakes. Tempeh is a traditional Indonesian food and remains a daily staple. Other grains are commonly combined with soybeans to make tempeh. Look for soy tempeh, which contains more soy protein than other varieties.

Tempeh is usually found in the refrigerator or freezer section of grocery stores. It can be kept at home in the refrigerator for about ten days or in the freezer for several months.

Miso

Miso is a rich, flavorful paste made from fermented, aged whole soybeans. It has a distinctive flavor and is used primarily as a soup base in several Asian cultures. Miso is available in Asian markets and well-stocked grocery stores and keeps well in the refrigerator for several months.

Soy Milk

Soy milk, sometimes called soy drink or soy beverage, is the liquid made from cooked soybeans that have been soaked, then ground and strained. Nonfat varieties are available. Several flavored drinks or beverages made from soy milk are also available. Check the label; some of these have sugar, corn syrup, or other sweeteners or flavorings added. Most of the recipes in this book use plain, nonfat soy milk.

You will find soy milk in most grocery stores, usually in shelf-stable single-serving or quart containers. Once it is opened, it must be stored in the refrigerator and should be used within a week. It is also available as a powder, which is reconstituted with water.

Soy Flour

Soy flour is made from hulled roasted soybeans that have been ground into a fine powder. It is available full-fat or defatted, which has the oils removed during processing and is higher in soy protein. Soy flour has a pleasant texture and a nutty flavor, which can be enhanced by lightly toasting it. Baked products containing soy flour tend to brown quickly, so baking time is shorter than for products made with wheat flour.

Soy flour is available in stores where grains and legumes are sold in bulk and in well-stocked grocery stores. Store it in a tightly covered container in the refrigerator.

Soy Protein Powder

Soy protein powder is made from defatted soybean flakes. It has the highest concentration of protein (90 percent) of all soy products because it is essentially all protein. You can buy it in stores where grains and legumes are sold in bulk. Many products are available that contain soy protein powder mixed with other ingredients such as sugar or other carbohydrates, flavorings, fillers, and additives that lower the protein content. Our recipes use plain soy protein powder, which is available in bulk for three to five dollars a pound.

Soy Sauce

Most Americans are familiar with soy sauce, which is made from fermented soybeans and used to flavor many Asian foods. Soy sauce usually contains wheat as well as soy. Tamari soy sauce, which we use in these recipes, is made exclusively from soybeans. Most people are aware that soy sauce is high in sodium. However, using a small amount of a flavorful quality sauce like tamari can reduce sodium intake. Remember, though, that soy sauce does not count as part of your soy intake, since it has no known health benefits.

FLAX

Flaxseed is the richest known plant source of omega-3 fatty acids and weak estrogens, making it a potential superfood. A new Canadian study found that 50 grams of ground flaxseed a day could "slow down tumor growth." First cited in the *Breast Cancer Prevention Diet* book three years ago, these researchers have now expanded their work to fifty women recently diagnosed with breast cancer and presented their findings at an international breast cancer conference in San Antonio, Texas, in December 2000. While waiting for surgery, these women were divided into two separate groups. Group one received 50 grams of ground flaxseed, eaten in a daily muffin. Group two ate the muffin, but it contained no flaxseed. At the time of surgery, those who had eaten the flaxseed had slower-growing tumors. This work has encouraged many women to incorporate flaxseed into their daily diet as a way of decreasing their risk of breast cancer, on the assumption that if it can shrink an existing breast tumor, it may play a powerful role in slowing the growth of microscopic tumors. You should discuss with your doctor if this is a useful strategy for you. If it is, here's how you can add this benefit to your daily diet. First, you'll need to grind your flaxseed to break down the seeds' hard outer coat, using a coffee-bean grinder. You can then add this to many of the items in your daily menu: orange juice, yogurt, muffins, breads, cereals, cottage cheese — even sprinkle some on your salad. You won't need special recipes to incorporate flaxseed into your meal plans, and the crunchy feel and nutty taste add extra zest to your foods. Be aware that flaxseed oil doesn't have these benefits.

FATS

Asian women eat dramatically less fat than Americans, with fat accounting for as little as 10 percent of their total calorie intake. Many doctors believe it's a safe bet to mirror Asian women's fat intake. The link to breast cancer in American women, however, is not proven, so the menu plans in this book allow you to choose meals containing as little as 15 percent of calories from fat in the New American and Asian meal plans and as much as 25 percent of calories from fat in the Mediterranean plan. The average fat intake in the United States is about 40 percent of total calories. If you have a high risk for breast cancer, as identified by a strong family history, you may want to choose the lowest-fat meal plans. We have reduced the fat in the menu plans in our book by selecting foods that are naturally low in fat and using preparation methods requiring very little added fat.

Fat makes food taste good. However, a little can go a long way, as you will see in our recipes. Many of our recipes have just a few drops of a flavored oil to enhance the food. Fat also makes you feel full. Again, including just a small amount of fat will make you feel satisfied at the end of the meal. In our recipes, the small amount of fat that is used, from olive and canola oils, is rich in monounsaturated fatty acids. For healthy breasts, the kind of fat you use is quite important. Olive oil is the healthiest you can use in cooking.

CRUCIFEROUS VEGETABLES

Cruciferous vegetables get their name from the branching (crosslike) stems they all have in common. Examples include broccoli, cauliflower, and cabbage. One study found that European women who ate more cabbage had a lower breast cancer death rate. In a study in Wisconsin, cruciferous vegetables decreased the risk of breast cancer by 40 percent.

HOW CRUCIFEROUS VEGETABLES WORK
TO PREVENT BREAST CANCER

There are "good" estrogens and "bad" estrogens, just as there are good and bad cholesterols. The *Journal of the National Cancer Institute* reported that the "bad" estrogen may be a factor in breast cancer development in Finnish women, since it permanently binds to the estrogen receptor. This receptor is on the breast duct cell, the cell most likely to become cancerous. That's like pressing a car horn and releasing the pressure only to find that it's stuck. All other estrogens attach briefly and then are released. Bad estrogen also causes mutations in breast cells. Women with breast cancer have almost twice as much bad estrogen as those without.

Only one family of vegetables increases the amount of good estrogen while decreasing the bad. Their special ingredient is called indole-3-carbinol.

The following are vegetables containing indole-3-carbinol:

- *Bitter cress*
- *Bok choy*
- *Broccoli*
- *Brussels sprouts*
- *Cabbage*
- *Cauliflower*
- *Collard*
- *Horseradish*
- *Kale*
- *Mustard seed*
- *Radishes*
- *Rutabaga (swede)*
- *Savoy cabbage*
- *Turnip*
- *Watercress*

SUPERTASTERS

Don't like cruciferous vegetables? Little wonder. You are one of what scientists call a supertaster, a person who finds these vegetables taste unusually bitter. Researchers believe that you are at a genetic disadvantage because you won't eat the vegetables that have the most powerful cancer-fighting effect. I've got to admit I'm one. I've never liked these vegetables and neither does my family. I do like fresh broccoli, not the limp, steamed kind. Coleslaw may be the most palatable choice of cruciferous vegetable for you, if it's made with the right low-fat dressing.

The lunch and dinner menus in this book contain at least one serving of cruciferous vegetables. The recipes in this book provide examples of different ways to prepare and use cruciferous vegetables to allow the characteristic flavors to stand out boldly and complement the other foods in the meal. We hope you'll be pleasantly surprised at how good they taste and trust that cruciferous vegetables will soon be among your favorites.

CONSUMER TIPS

The active ingredient indole-3-carbinol can be deactivated by heat. For that reason you'll want to avoid badly wilted cruciferous vegetables. Lightly steaming or stir-frying them can maintain the active ingredient.

WHOLE GRAINS

Large amounts of refined flours in the food can raise blood insulin levels. In a study of 535 breast cancer patients followed for as long as ten years, those with the highest insulin levels were more than eight times more likely to die than women with the lowest insulin levels. And they were almost four times as likely to have their cancer recur at a distant site.

Dr. Pamela J. Goodwin of the University of Toronto presented these findings at the May 2000 annual meeting of the American Society of Clinical Oncology. High insulin levels also increase your risk of obesity and type II diabetes.

Choose whole-grain breads, cereals, and pastas over refined flours, pasta, white rice, and potatoes.

FORTIFIED CEREALS

Breast cancer rates vary directly with the amount of solar radiation. The colder, cloudier Northeast has a higher rate of breast cancer than the warmer, sunnier south. What's the connection? Exposure to sunlight helps the body manufacture vitamin D. Vitamin D is a potent inhibitor of a cell's ability to divide and grow. Vitamin D also helps breast cells to become more mature so they are less vulnerable to cancer-causing toxins. Fortified cereals are an excellent source of vitamin D and form the core of a healthy breakfast, as are dairy products.

FRESH FRUITS AND VEGETABLES

The menu plans in this book are high in fruits and vegetables, containing an average of nine to eleven servings, including two servings of cruciferous vegetables a day. This is considerably more than the average of three to four servings of fruits and vegetables that most Americans eat.

Fruits and vegetables bring an incredibly rich palette of colors, textures, and tastes to the American table. They are available in great variety and abundance to enjoy year-round. People who eat them every day are healthier than those who don't. Fruits and vegetables are rich sources of compounds such as fiber, antioxidants, vitamins, minerals, and phytochemicals that have been shown to prevent cancer and other chronic diseases. Their greatest importance in breast cancer prevention is their potential to stifle the cellular mechanisms that initiate cancer.

The American Institute of Cancer Research (AICR) recently reported that diets containing substantial amounts of a variety of vegetables and fruits will help reduce the risk in 20 percent or more of all cases of cancer. Eating sufficient fruits and vegetables has also been associated with reduced rates of heart disease, stroke, high blood pressure, birth defects, chronic diseases of the gastrointestinal tract, and even cataracts. Scientific research continues to support the positive role of fruits and vegetables in long-term health. Despite the luxurious year-round availability of fruits and vegetables and the mounting evidence of their role in promoting health and preventing disease, the fruit and vegetable intake of many Americans is surprisingly low. Consider this, however: the fruits and vegetables that are richest in cancer-fighting antioxidants are often the tastiest. For instance, kale and sweet potatoes are among the highest-ranked vegetables, while cantaloupe and strawberries lead the list of best fruits.

Each culture has its own distinctive fruits and vegetables that reflect the agricultural conditions and climate of the region. Because of technological advances in growing, harvesting, and transporting produce, the worldwide market of fruits and vegetables is constantly expanding. Each of the three types of menu plans presented in the next chapter highlights the unique fruits and vegetables of the region. Choose fresh, locally grown produce as much as possible.

FIBER

Fiber traps estrogen in the intestine so that it is not recirculated into the bloodstream. This reduces the amount of estrogen in the bloodstream that can reach the breast. The menu plans in this book contain about 35 grams of total dietary fiber a day. Most people in America get a lot less than that, only about 10 to 12 grams a day.

Fiber is found in legumes such as soybeans and other beans, lentils, whole grains, and fruits and vegetables. As you can see, foods that are good sources of fiber are usually sources of other protective nutrients as well. We recommend getting your fiber from a variety of foods that provide these protective nutrients rather than from supplements or from only one food source. The easiest way to increase your fiber intake is by eating a cup or so of beans a day and a bowl of high-fiber breakfast cereal.

Scientific research is still identifying and classifying types of fiber in foods. Currently, dietary fiber is classified as either soluble or insoluble. Foods rich in soluble fiber include oats, apples, oranges, carrots, beans and other legumes, and dried fruits. Foods rich in insoluble fiber include wheat bran, whole grains, fruits, and vegetables. Soluble and insoluble fibers have different health-promoting effects in the body. Therefore it's best to include food sources of both types every day. The menu plans in this book have been designed to provide generous amounts of both soluble and insoluble fiber.

A word of caution: In some individuals an abrupt increase in high-fiber foods may cause general intestinal discomfort such as bloating. If your usual eating plan doesn't include legumes, whole grains, and fruits and vegetables, increase your consumption gradually, adding one of these foods a day so that you can gradually adjust to a higher fiber intake. And be sure to drink lots of water, at least six to eight glasses a day.

PLANNING FOR CHANGE

Depending on your current habits, this eating plan may or may not be a radical departure from your usual way of eating. It might be helpful for you to keep a food record for a few days before you begin. Write down everything you eat and drink. Evaluate your current eating plan to identify the positive things you are already doing that you should continue. For instance, are you getting lots of fruits and vegetables? Do you choose whole-grain products most of the time? If so, you will be continuing these practices and building on them through our menus.

If you are not currently eating sufficient quantities of the foods mentioned above, then gradually introduce menus from any of the three meal plans. Most of us have ten favorite meals. If you can learn to shop for, cook, and enjoy even ten new meals, you'll go a long way toward making yourself the healthiest you've ever been. By making these changes, you will have optimized your chances of preventing cancer and other chronic diseases and done your best. It is our hope that you will enjoy the foods, the meal plans, and a new way of eating.

Nutrition is an art and a science, and you'll find the best of both here. This book brings you the art of nutrition by creating appetizing meals that you will find irresistible; it brings the science of nutrition by creating meals that have been planned to provide the specific combinations of nutrients that are most protective of the breast.

NUTRITION INFORMATION

Each meal has been carefully analyzed for key nutrients to be certain you are at least getting adequate amounts. You'll find the nutrient content of the key nutrients at the end of each recipe.

TERMS

Below is a list of cooking terms used in this book and how we define them.

Baste: To periodically spoon or brush liquid over food while cooking, to keep it moist and add flavor.

Blanch: To immerse briefly in boiling water. To blanch a food, bring a large quantity of water (enough to hold the food without crowding) to boiling. Add the food; continue heating over high heat until the water returns to a boil. Drain and rinse immediately under cold running water. Blanching intensifies the color and texture of a food.

Cooking time: The time it takes for the final cooking of the dish once all the ingredients are prepared.

Marinades: Richly flavored liquids that tenderize and enhance the flavor of meats and vegetables. Sometimes marinades are used as the base for a sauce accompanying a dish.

Mince: To chop into very small pieces.

Preparation time: The amount of time needed to gather the ingredients in the kitchen and prepare them for the recipe. This includes washing fruits and vegetables, chopping or slicing foods, and sautéing or roasting ingredients for use in a recipe. The time listed is approximate.

Sauté: To brown in a small amount of fat, generally in a frying pan.

Simmer: To heat liquid just below the boiling point. To simmer a liquid, bring it to a boil, then immediately adjust the heat so that small bubbles break just along the rim of the pan.

Steam: To cook food in steam over boiling water in a closed container. If you don't have a steamer, you can use a small metal or wooden rack in a saucepan with a tight-fitting lid, keeping the water level below the rack.

Steep: To let foods stand in a liquid below boiling point, Steeping is used to extract flavor and/or color from a food.

Stir-fry: To fry thinly sliced foods quickly in only a little oil, stirring constantly.

Stock: Water flavored by the specific ingredients that are cooked in it. It is used as the base for soups, stews, and sauces.

Toast: To heat nuts to brown them and intensify their flavor. To toast nuts, preheat the oven to 300 degrees. Spread nuts on a cookie sheet and place in the preheated oven for about 5 minutes, turning frequently. Nuts burn quickly when they are heated, so watch them carefully to avoid burning. Just a few toasted nuts will add wonderful flavor to many recipes. Toasted nuts retain their crispness and flavor when stored in a sealed container in the refrigerator.

CONVERSION TABLE

For your convenience, here is a table with common weights and measures:

Volume

3 teaspoons = 1 tablespoon
2 tablespoons = 1 fluid ounce
4 tablespoons = ¼ cup
5⅓ tablespoons = ⅓ cup
8 tablespoons = ½ cup
16 tablespoons = 1 cup
2 cups = 1 pint
2 pints = 1 quart
4 quarts = 1 gallon

Weight

16 ounces = 1 pound

OTHER TERMS

Phytochemicals: Substances found in fruits, vegetables, and legumes that exert a biochemical effect having the potential to prevent cancer.

Antioxidants: Substances that protect healthy cells against unstable oxygen molecules in the body. Some examples of antioxidants are beta-carotene, vitamins C and E, and lycopene.

SHOPPING

The recipes and menu ideas in this book are based on whole, fresh foods as much as possible. I live in Manhattan, while Rita and Barbara live in the San Francisco Bay area. We're all blessed with an abundance of fresh produce all year long. There are many markets featuring exotic varieties of produce. It's not unusual for a well-stocked market to offer more than ten varieties of apples or tomatoes, for instance. The ethnic diversity of both areas guarantees that there are produce markets, delis, and grocery stores featuring foods that are not commonly available in some areas of the United States.

Since not everyone has access to this diverse, plentiful supply of foods, we decided to limit the ingredients used in the recipes to those most likely to be available in well-stocked grocery stores everywhere. If an item is not available, request that the store manager stock it. We encourage you to patronize local farmers markets for really fresh fruits and vegetables at their prime. You'll taste the difference that freshness makes! Remember to wash all produce well to remove dirt and grit, as well as possible pesticides and herbicides.

A NOTE ON COST

When you first stock your pantry with the items you'll need for the Asian, New American, and Mediterranean menus, you might find that you've spent a lot of money on sauces, vinegars, oils, and spices. This money is well spent, since you can enjoy these ingredients for years to come.

Let's now look in on three fabulous lifestyles and the cuisines they fostered, from the exotic lands of the Far East to the lush shores of the Mediterranean Sea to the fabled wine country of the Napa Valley of California. In each of these cuisines are the secrets of a long and healthy life and the promise of a formidable weapon against the beginnings of breast cancer.

THE MENU PLANS

ASIAN MENU PLANS

The term *Asian food* encompasses the cuisines of many ancient cultures. The cooking of each country reflects the predominant availability of certain foods. There is the use of coconut milk and red chilies in Thailand, the liberal use of fish in the island country of Japan, and the seasonal vegetables used in the satisfying Vietnamese noodle soup pho, commonly served at breakfast. Even within countries, there are regionally distinct cuisines characterized by the use of local foods, seasonal produce, and unique blends of spices.

Although there are differences, there are also many similarities among Asian cuisines: among them, the use of rice or noodles as the staple of each meal, the use of fresh ingredients whenever possible, and the inclusion of some form of soy. Traditional foods still predominate in Asia, and even in the far-flung communities of the diaspora, these ingredients continue to be staples.

In the menu plans for this section, we used rice or noodles as the staple of each meal. We have substituted brown rice for the traditional white rice staple in order to achieve adequate fiber intake. To make these meals even healthier, you can also use wild rice and whole-grain noodles. We used fresh ingredients and chose them carefully for a balance of flavor, color, and texture of the dish. We also used soy with most meals.

Some flavors are ubiquitous in Asian cooking — ginger, garlic, mushrooms, carrots, bok choy, onions, and lychees. We have incorporated these flavors throughout our menu plans.

You might be surprised to find soup or rice and vegetables for breakfast. Some Asian cultures don't have specific foods for different meals; breakfast may include flavorful soup or leftover vegetables served with rice.

Since coconut milk, an ingredient in a couple of the recipes in this section, is usually very high in fat, we made our own. The recipe on page 221 has all the flavor of the traditional coconut milk but none of the fat.

The Asian menus contain whole grains and eleven servings of fruits and vegetables a day, including two cruciferous vegetables. They are low in fat (15 percent of total calories) and have approximately 35 grams of total dietary fiber a day. The Asian menus provide adequate amounts of protein, vitamins, and minerals.

The Asian menus are rich in soy protein, providing an estimated 35 grams a day — approximately 19 grams come from the meals and an additional 16 grams from your daily shake.

BREAST-HEALTHY SOY PROTEIN SHAKE

This shake provides 16 grams of soy protein. It is an excellent, nutritious afternoon pick-me-up. If you like, have half a recipe for a midmorning or nighttime snack and the other half for an afternoon snack.

You may substitute other fruits for the banana and strawberries. For a thicker shake, freeze the fruit ahead of time.

YIELD: 1 SERVING

PREPARATION TIME: 5 MINUTES

COOKING TIME: NONE

INGREDIENTS:

1 cup nonfat milk
2 tablespoons packed soy protein powder
1 tablespoon orange juice concentrate
½ medium banana, cut in chunks
½ cup strawberries

Put all ingredients in a blender. Blend until smooth.

Estimated nutrients per serving:
Calories: 240
Total protein (grams): 26
Soy protein (grams): 16
Total carbohydrate (grams): 34
Total fat (grams): 2
Total fiber (grams): 3
Total fruit and vegetable (servings): 1

PROSTATE PROTECTION NOTE

Asian meals for prostate cancer prevention are extremely low in fat (10 percent of total calories from fat), and have NO dairy or other animal products. If you're cooking for men in your household who are trying to protect themselves from prostate cancer, the Asian meal plans best satisfy the stringent requirements of a prostate-specific eating plan. The Mediterranean and New American recipes are quite beneficial for men at lower risk of prostate cancer but contain more fat than men at the very highest risk should be eating.

You can use most recipes in the menus starting on page 29 for prostate cancer protection without modifying them; necessary alterations are given at the end of the recipe. The recipes themselves outline how you would change the ingredients for prostate health.

Here are two easy ways to include prostate-healthy foods in your diet:

1. Serve one 6-ounce glass of canned tomato juice with a meal every day.
2. Serve one Prostate-Healthy Soy Protein Shake a day.

PROSTATE-HEALTHY SOY PROTEIN SHAKE

This is an adaptation of the Breast-Healthy Soy Protein Shake and is made with nonfat soy milk instead of regular nonfat milk, giving it 4 more grams of soy protein.

YIELD: 1 SERVING

PREPARATION TIME: 5 MINUTES

COOKING TIME: NONE

INGREDIENTS:

1 cup nonfat soy milk
2 tablespoons packed soy protein powder
1 tablespoon orange juice concentrate
½ medium banana, cut in chunks
½ cup strawberries

Put all ingredients in a blender. Blend until smooth.

Estimated nutrients per serving:
Calories: 240
Total protein (grams): 26
Soy protein (grams): 20
Total carbohydrate (grams): 34
Total fat (grams): 2
Total fiber (grams): 3
Total fruit and vegetable (servings): 1

Note: *The shake for breast cancer is made with nonfat cow's milk. Women need calcium to prevent osteoporosis, so we used cow's milk to ensure adequate calcium. The shake for prostate cancer is made with soy milk instead of cow's milk, resulting in 20 grams of soy protein.*

THE WELL-STOCKED ASIAN PANTRY

ON THE SHELF:

Asian-style vermicelli noodles
bamboo shoots
black bean sauce
brown rice
canned mandarin oranges
canola oil
chili oil
dried black mushrooms
fish sauce
hoisin sauce (a rich brown sauce used extensively in Asian cooking because of its distinctive sweet, spicy flavor)
lychees
mature soybeans

mirin (a sweet cooking sake)
miso
orange-blossom water
prepared black soybeans
red pepper flakes
rice noodles
rice vinegar
sesame oil
sherry vinegar
tamari soy sauce
water chestnuts

IN THE REFRIGERATOR:

baby bok choy
baked tofu
broccoli
cabbage
carrots
cauliflower
cilantro
extra-firm tofu
fresh gingerroot*
fresh green soybeans
green onions
lemongrass
roasted garlic
silken tofu
soy tempeh

Note: We encourage the use of fresh produce whenever possible, so there is no list of freezer items. However, if you are pressed for time, some of these vegetables can be frozen.

---

* Our recipes use freshly grated gingerroot. Ginger stores well in the refrigerator. For best results, grate it just before using.

▪ ASIAN MENUS ▪

B R E A K F A S T

Soy Breakfast Smoothie, p. 47
Rice and Vegetables, p. 48

Tempeh with Snow Peas, Mushrooms, and Carrots, p. 49
Apple-Pear Slices

Vegetable Pho, p. 50
Sliced Orange

Griddle Rice Cakes, p. 51
with Curried Tofu, p. 52
Fresh Papaya and Mango Chutney, p. 120

Miso Soup, p. 53
Fresh Cherries and Mandarin Orange Slices

Enoki Mushroom Custard, p. 54
Crusty Whole Wheat Roll
Peach Slices

Crispy Noodles with Vegetables, p. 56
Banana

Grilled Marinated Mushrooms and Tomatoes, p. 57
Honeydew Melon Wedges

Egg Foo Yung, p. 58
Rice Wraps, p. 59
Kiwifruit (Chinese Gooseberries)

Asparagus and Carrot in Oyster Sauce, p. 61
Green Grapes

LUNCH

Tofu-Mushroom Soup, p. 91
Mixed Vegetable Stir-Fry, p. 123
Orange Slices in Orange Water, p. 222

Mu Shu Vegetables, p. 124
Carrot-Daikon Salad, p. 203
Asian Pear–Apple Slices

Broccoli-Mushroom Stir-Fry with Tofu, p. 125
Watercress Salad, p. 204
Kiwifruit and Pear Slices

Sweet and Sour Tofu, p. 127
Asparagus and Radish Salad, p. 204
Mandarin Orange Wedges

Vegetables and Tofu with Noodles, p. 128
Bean Sprout Salad, p. 205
Banana and Dried Cranberries

Tuna-Asparagus Salad, p. 166
French Bread
Fruit Jumble, p. 223

Black Mushroom Soup, p. 92
Fried Rice with Shrimp, p. 184
Lychees

Fresh Soybeans and Vegetables with Black Bean Sauce, p. 130
Celery and Water Chestnut Salad, p. 206
Guava Ice, p. 223

Spicy Noodle Salad, p. 167
Crusty Roll
Minted Melon, p. 224

Thai Soup, p. 93
Toasted Sesame Seed Baguette
Lychee Tapioca, p. 225

DINNER

Cauliflower and Carrot Curry with Tofu, p. 131
Mint Chutney, p. 121
Lychees and Mango Ice, p. 226

Laotian Fish Soup, p. 95
Pickled Cucumber and Onion, p. 207
Baked Banana in Orange Water, p. 227

Sweet and Sour Bok Choy and Tempeh, p. 132
Vietnamese Salad Rolls, p. 208
Mango Sorbet, p. 228

Grilled Fresh Tuna, p. 134
Fresh Vegetable Medley, p. 194
Papaya and Strawberries

Rice Noodles with Vegetables and Tofu in Black Bean Sauce, p. 135
Bean Sprout Salad, p. 205
Mung Bean Cake

Curried Soybeans and Broccoli, p. 136
Mint Chutney, p. 121
Indian Flatbread
Mango Lassi, p. 229

Tofu Kebobs, p. 137
Wilted Baby Bok Choy, p. 195
Fresh Papaya and Mango Chutney, p. 120
Fortune Cookies

Fish with Carrot and Broccoli in Plum Sauce, p. 139
Asparagus and Radish Salad, p. 204
Coconut Float, p. 230

Sweet and Sour Chicken, p. 140
Steamed Cauliflower and Fresh Soybeans, p. 196
Mandarin and Bing Cherry Tapioca, p. 231

Noodles with Celery, Carrot, and Broccoli, p. 141
Vietnamese Salad Rolls, p. 208
Poached Asian Pears, p. 232

NEW AMERICAN MENU PLANS

"American" cuisine started out as cooking for survival, adapting recipes from the Old World to indigenous fruits and vegetables. With modern transportation and technology, American cuisine has exploded, resulting in dishes still influenced by regional cultures but using the rich abundance of foods from the entire world.

From this vast cornucopia, we have selected foods with taste, health, and prevention of disease in mind. Traditional standbys, such as baked beans, macaroni and cheese, and burritos, have been modified to incorporate the nutritional elements of our preventive-eating plan while retaining their age-old appeal.

For the New American recipes, we have kept the use of traditional staples: fruits and vegetables, cereals and other grains, and beans. The cruciferous vegetables often include kale, collard greens, turnips, and rutabagas, in addition to the more widely used broccoli and cauliflower.

The importance of grains in the American cuisine is immortalized by the phrase "amber waves of grain" in the popular song "America the Beautiful." The abundant harvest of the Great Plains provides wheat and other whole grains, which are a veritable storehouse of nutrients. These grains provide a rich, flavorful background for the New American meals.

Soybeans and other beans and legumes are used as the main source of protein. They also provide other essential nutrients, including B vitamins, minerals, and fiber. In response to the increased demand of health-conscious consumers, a wider variety of beans is becoming available at local grocery stores. Some varieties of beans are available fresh, others dried or canned. Using canned beans in the recipes makes life easier for a busy cook. Some varieties of beans are only available dried. Be aware that dried beans can take several hours to cook and are best prepared a day ahead of time. See page 181 for cooking instructions. If you can't find the beans you're looking for in the grocery store, look in specialty-food stores where grains and legumes are sold in bulk.

The New American menus contain nine servings of fruits and vegetables a day, including two cruciferous vegetables. They are low in fat (15 percent of the total calories), are high in total dietary fiber (approximately 35 grams a day), and provide adequate amounts of carbohydrates, vitamins, and minerals. The menus also contain an estimated 35 grams of soy protein a day — approximately 19 grams come from the meals and an additional 16 grams from a shake (page 25). Don't forget to add this breast-healthy soy shake to your eating plan every day.

FOR PROSTATE PROTECTION

1. Drink one 6-ounce glass of canned tomato juice with a meal every day.

2. Make and drink one Prostate-Healthy Soy Protein Shake a day (page 26).

3. You can use most of the recipes in the menus starting on page 34 without modifying them. The recipes themselves outline how you would change the ingredients for prostate health.

THE WELL-STOCKED NEW AMERICAN PANTRY

ON THE SHELF:

balsamic vinegar
brown rice
bulgur (cracked wheat; see note on page 39)
canola oil
defatted soy flour
extra-light-taste olive oil (see note on page 39)
extra-virgin olive oil (see note on page 39)
lentils
nonfat soy milk
rolled oats
soy-protein powder
*steel-cut oats**
whole-wheat flour

---

* Steel-cut oats are often called coarse-cut oats, or simply oats. They are available in stores that sell grains in bulk.

IN THE REFRIGERATOR:

baby bok choy
baked tofu
broccoli
cabbage
cauliflower
collard greens
extra-firm tofu
kale
mature soybeans
nonfat plain yogurt
roasted garlic
rutabaga
silken tofu
soy tempeh
turnip

Note: *For maximum benefit, buy fresh produce. However, any of the vegetables listed above may be purchased frozen, if available.*
Homemade vegetable or fish stock may be frozen for later use.

▪ NEW AMERICAN MENUS ▪

BREAKFAST

Homemade Muesli, p. 63
Orange Slices
Grapefruit Juice

Steel-Cut Oatmeal with Sun-Dried Cranberries and Walnuts, p. 64
Orange Juice

Eggs Florentine, p. 65
Seven-Grain Bread
Apple-Cranberry Juice

Buckwheat Pancakes with Berries, p. 66
Mango-Guava Nectar

All-Bran Cereal with Soy Milk and Banana
Pineapple Juice

Crunchy Homemade Granola, p. 67
Soy Milk
Orange Juice

Super Toast with Ginger Yogurt, p. 69
Orange-Pineapple Juice

Date-Orange Muffins, p. 70
Pear Juice

Rye Bagel with Savory Spread, p. 71
Tomato Juice

Coffee Cake, p. 72
Nonfat Vanilla Yogurt
Orange Juice

LUNCH

Vegetable-Potato Salad, p. 169
Sesame Seed Roll
Kiwifruit

Bean and Broccoli Burrito with Tomato-Corn Salsa, p. 143
Strawberry and Orange Fruit Plate

Kale and Cucumber Soup, p. 97
Whole Wheat Bran Roll
Lemon-Raspberry Sorbet, p. 234

Open-Face Lentil-Nut Loaf Sandwich, p. 111
Fresh Spinach and Red Cabbage Salad, p. 210
Dried Fig Slices and Nonfat Vanilla Yogurt

Spring Artichoke Heart Salad, p. 170
Low-Fat Whole Wheat Crackers
Mandarin Orange Wedges

Salmon Luncheon Salad, p. 171
Crusty Roll
Apple and Pear Slices

Smoked Tofu Sandwich, p. 112
Radish Slices and Broccoli Florets
Fresh Melon Slices

Tuna Melt, p. 114
Garden Salad, p. 210
Oatmeal Cookies, p. 235

Baked Beans, p. 144
Healthy Coleslaw, p. 211
Corn Bread, p. 186
Apple Wedges

Macaroni and Cheese, p. 145
Steamed Broccoli and Red Pepper Rings
Grape Clusters

DINNER

Black Bean and Mushroom Stew with Parmesan Polenta, p. 98
Steamed Broccoli
Garden Salad, p. 210
Peach Slices and Raspberries with Lemon Sherbet

Grilled Swordfish with Roasted Corn and Red Pepper Salsa, p. 146
Quinoa, p. 187
Lemon Carrots and Collard Greens, p. 197
Crusty Dinner Roll
Ginger Yogurt, p. 236

Three-Bean Chili, p. 100
Warmed Whole Wheat Tortillas
Mixed Greens and Tomato Salad, p. 212
Honeydew Melon and Blueberries

Black Bean and Rice Soup, p. 101
Crusty French Bread
Spinach and Orange Salad, p. 213
Fresh Figs and Walnuts with Vanilla Topping, p. 237

Stuffed Red Pepper, p. 148
Steamed Fresh Asparagus
Grainy Whole Wheat Roll
Baked Apples with Vanilla Yogurt, p. 238

Cottage Pie, p. 149
Whole Steamed String Beans
Spring Greens, p. 214
Poached Pears with Nutmeg Topping, p. 239

Grilled Salmon with Sesame and Lime, p. 150
Mixed-Grain Pilaf, p. 188
Steamed Broccoli
Chocolate Pudding, p. 240

Spaghetti with Tomato-Tempeh Sauce, p. 151
Green Salad, p. 214
Italian Bread
Strawberry Frozen Dessert, p. 241

English Chicken-Mushroom Casserole, p. 153
Steamed Kale, p. 192
Tapioca Pudding, p. 242

Fajitas, p. 154
Green Salad, p. 214
Fruit Compote, p. 243

MEDITERRANEAN MENU PLANS

Mediterranean conjures up images of sunshine, the azure sea, hills ter-
raced with olive trees, and a lust for life, which includes the enjoyment
of food. Bountiful summertime harvests provide a wide variety of re-

gional foods, including olives, garlic, peppers, artichokes, eggplants, grapes, figs, dates, lemons, oranges, and nuts. We used these foods as the foundation of our menu plans. The recipes in the book are modifications of popular dishes from countries of the Mediterranean region, including Italy, Greece, Spain, France, Turkey, and Morocco.

In the Mediterranean region, desserts are often simple. The food-loving people of this region often prefer to end a meal with luscious fresh fruits and ices. We have chosen to incorporate this practice in our Mediterranean menu plans.

The "Mediterranean diet" has received some attention in recent years and is promoted to be associated with longevity. Although there are several variations, the core components include a high consumption of olive oil, fruits and vegetables, legumes, and grains; a moderate consumption of milk and other dairy products and wine; and a low consumption of meat and meat products.

The Mediterranean menu plans in this book are similar in that they are high in fruits, vegetables, legumes, and grains. However, our menu plans differ in that soy is used as the main protein source in place of dairy products and meat, and olive oil is used in moderate amounts.

The menus contain eleven servings of fruits and vegetables a day, including two cruciferous vegetables. They are moderate in fat, containing 25 percent of the calories from fat, mostly olive oil. Because of the inclusion of whole grains, fruits, vegetables, and legumes, they are high in total dietary fiber, containing approximately 35 grams a day. In addition, the Mediterranean menus provide adequate amounts of carbohydrate, vitamins, and minerals. The menus contain an estimated 35 grams of soy protein a day — approximately 19 grams come from the meals and an additional 16 grams from our soy shake (page 25).

FOR PROSTATE PROTECTION

1. Drink one 6-ounce glass of canned tomato juice with a meal every day.
2. Make and drink one Prostate-Healthy Soy Protein Shake a day (page 26).
3. You can use most of the recipes in the menus starting on page 40 without modifying them. The recipes themselves outline how you would change the ingredients for prostate health.

THE WELL-STOCKED MEDITERRANEAN PANTRY

ON THE SHELF:

almonds
black olives
brown rice
*bulgur (cracked wheat)**
couscous†
dates
dried figs
extra-light-taste olive oil‡
extra-virgin olive oil‡
nonfat soy milk
soy protein powder
whole wheat flour

IN THE REFRIGERATOR:

baby bok choy
broccoli
cabbage
cauliflower
eggplant
fresh green soybeans
green bell peppers
nonfat plain yogurt
orange juice

---

* Bulgur is whole wheat that has been prepared by boiling and drying. It is dehydrated and needs to be soaked in water before use. Bulgur has the delicate, nutty flavor of a whole grain.

† Couscous gets its name from the Arabic word for semolina, which is milled from durum wheat. This tiny pasta is prepared by soaking in hot water for five minutes.

‡ The process of pressing olives results in oils that vary from extra-virgin to extra-light. The nutritional value of all these is the same. The terms refer to differences in taste, color, and aroma, as follows:

 ■ Extra-virgin olive oil results from the first "press" of cold olives. It is darker than other olive oils. Extra-virgin olive oil is very flavorful and is best used when you want this flavor as part of the dish, such as in salads and pasta dishes.

 ■ At the other end of the spectrum is extra-light-taste olive oil. When used with olive oil, the term *extra-light* refers to the taste, not fat content, as it does on most food labels. Extra-light-taste olive oil is pale green in color with a light olive flavor. Use it as a general cooking oil when you don't want the strong flavor of olive oil to permeate the dish.

oranges
peaches
roasted garlic
rutabaga
savory baked tofu
silken tofu
soy tempeh
sweet red peppers

■ MEDITERRANEAN MENUS ■

BREAKFAST

Goat Cheese with Melon and Figs, p. 74
Toasted Dense Whole Wheat Bread
Orange Juice

Artichoke Frittata, p. 74
Baked Roma Tomatoes with Fresh Basil, p. 198
Black Olive Focaccia
Grapefruit Juice

Cornmeal Waffles with Peaches and Berries, p. 76
Pineapple Juice

Buckwheat Crepes with Date-Orange Filling, p. 77
Strawberry-Guava Nectar

Peach-Orange Smoothie, p. 78
Toasted Whole Wheat Nut Bread

Savory Breakfast Roll, p. 79
Apple Slices
Pineapple-Orange Juice

Couscous with Dried Fruit and Almonds, p. 81
Cranapple Juice

Date Breakfast Bars, p. 82
Grilled Grapefruit Half, p. 83
Pear Nectar

Olive Soda Bread, p. 84
Slices of Roma Tomato and Low-Fat Mozzarella Cheese
Apple Juice

Citrus Delight, p. 85
Breakfast Aram, p. 86
Pineapple-Orange-Banana Juice

LUNCH

Pita Bread Sandwich, p. 116
Roma Tomatoes with Olive Oil, p. 216
Fuji Apple Slices and Figs

Minestrone, p. 103
Whole Wheat Focaccia
Bosc Pear Slices

Spring Cracked Wheat Salad, p. 173
Crisp Bread Sticks
Sliced Kiwifruit and Banana

Greek Sandwich, p. 117
Broccoli Salad, p. 217
Strawberries

Roasted Peppers and Eggplant Salad, p. 174
Flatbread
with Soybean Hummus, p. 182
Plums

White Bean Stew, p. 104
Pita Bread
Fresh Peach Slices
with Ginger Yogurt, p. 236

Aram Sandwich, p. 118
Sweet Red and Green Bell Pepper Strips
Fresh Bing Cherries

Potato-Kale Soup, p. 105
Whole Wheat Baguette
Bartlett Pear Slices and Ruby Grapes

Antipasto, p. 175
Marinated Cauliflower, p. 217
French Bread
Kumquat Halves and Kiwi Slices

Vegetable and Barley Salad, p. 176
Parmesan Cheese Bread Sticks
Lemon Sorbet with Marie Biscuits

DINNER

Vegetable and Bean Ragout over Couscous, p. 106
Field Greens, p. 218
Apple and Grapefruit Slices with Currants

Green Cabbage Stuffed with Bulgur and Vegetables, p. 156
Baked Roma Tomatoes with Fresh Basil, p. 198
Whole Wheat Roll
Fresh Strawberries with Lemon Sorbet

Bouillabaisse, p. 108
French Bread
Romaine with Balsamic Vinegar Dressing, p. 200
Mixed Berry Ice, p. 245

Ratatouille, p. 109
Soft Bread Sticks
Spinach and Orange Salad, p. 213
Minted Melon Slices, p. 246

Linguine with Lentils, p. 157
Steamed French Green Beans
Hearty Bread
Plums with Yogurt, p. 247

Swordfish Kebobs, p. 159
Rice and Kale Pilaf, p. 190
Steamed Carrot Coins
Citrus-Spritzed Strawberries, p. 247

Lasagna, p. 160
Italian Bread
Spinach and Grated-Carrot Salad, p. 219
Barbara's Orange Dessert, p. 248

Kubbul, p. 161
Salad with Capers, p. 220
Melon, Raspberry, and Cherry Cocktail, p. 249

Baked Trout Fillets, p. 163
Sautéed Soybeans, p. 191
Steamed Brussels Sprouts
Dinner Roll
Cheese Tart with Kiwi and Strawberries, p. 250

Tricolor Pasta with Tomato and Soybean Sauce, p. 164
Sicilian Cabbage, p. 199
Crusty French Bread
Nectarine Slices and Green Grapes

PART II

RECIPES

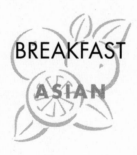

BREAKFAST

SOY BREAKFAST SMOOTHIE

Be creative and try adding about half a cup of fruit or combinations of fruits, such as strawberries and kiwifruit or peaches and raspberries. If the fruit is fresh or canned (drain the liquid), put pieces of fruit on a tray in the freezer and freeze until firm before adding them to the smoothie.

YIELD: 1 SERVING

PREPARATION TIME: 5 MINUTES

COOKING TIME: NONE

INGREDIENTS:

1 cup nonfat soy milk
1 tablespoon frozen orange juice concentrate
1 tablespoon soy protein powder
½ large banana, frozen
¼ teaspoon vanilla flavoring
3 ice cubes, crushed
Sprinkle grated nutmeg

1. Put all ingredients except nutmeg in a blender. Blend until smooth.
2. Pour into a glass, sprinkle with nutmeg.

Estimated nutrients per serving:

Calories: 240
Total protein (grams): 15
Soy protein (grams): 14
Total carbohydrate (grams): 45
Total fat (grams): 1

Total fiber (grams): 4
Total fruit and vegetable (servings): 1

For prostate protection: *You can use this recipe as is.*

RICE AND VEGETABLES

This easy-to-prepare breakfast is a great way to begin a day with a full work schedule.

YIELD: 2 SERVINGS
PREPARATION TIME: 10 MINUTES
COOKING TIME: 10 MINUTES

INGREDIENTS:

2 teaspoons canola oil
8 small shiitake mushrooms, sliced
12 thin asparagus spears, tough ends removed, cut diagonally
16 pieces bamboo shoots
1 teaspoon freshly grated ginger
6 drops chili oil
2 cups cooked brown rice (page 178)

1. In a medium skillet or wok, heat canola oil over medium-high heat.
2. Add mushrooms, asparagus, bamboo shoots, and ginger. Cook for 5 minutes, stirring frequently.
3. Add chili oil and stir.
4. Serve over brown rice.

Estimated nutrients per serving:

Calories: 290
Total protein (grams): 8
Soy protein (grams): 0
Total carbohydrate (grams): 51
Total fat (grams): 7
Total fiber (grams): 5
Total fruit and vegetable (servings): 2

For prostate protection: *You can use this recipe as is.*

TEMPEH WITH SNOW PEAS, MUSHROOMS, AND CARROTS

The rich and interesting aromas of this dish whet your appetite while you prepare it. The distinctive background flavor comes from the hoisin sauce, mirin, and fresh ginger.

YIELD: 2 SERVINGS
PREPARATION TIME: 10 MINUTES
COOKING TIME: 5 MINUTES

INGREDIENTS:
1 teaspoon hoisin sauce
1 teaspoon mirin
¼ teaspoon freshly grated ginger
¼ cup water
4 ounces soy tempeh, sliced
¼ teaspoon canola oil
1 small carrot, thinly sliced on the diagonal
2 medium green onions, including the green top, sliced
2 large mushrooms, sliced
10 medium snow peas, thinly sliced on the diagonal
2 cups cooked brown rice (page 178)

1. In a medium bowl, combine the hoisin sauce, mirin, ginger, and water. Add the tempeh and stir gently until marinade covers the tempeh. Set aside.
2. In a medium nonstick skillet, heat the oil over medium-high heat. Add carrot and green onions; sauté for 1 minute. Add mushrooms and snow peas; continue sautéing for another minute.
3. Add tempeh and marinade. Heat and stir until the sauce comes to a boil.
4. Serve over brown rice.

Estimated nutrients per serving:
Calories: 390
Total protein (grams): 18
Soy protein (grams): 11
Total carbohydrate (grams): 61
Total fat (grams): 7

Total fiber (grams): 11
Total fruit and vegetable (servings): 2

For prostate protection: *To increase lycopene, add ¼ cup of tomato puree to the hoisin sauce mixture.*

VEGETABLE PHO

Pho is a staple of Vietnamese cuisine and is commonly eaten at breakfast. A full-bodied broth flavor is crucial to pho. The broth can be made ahead in quantity to have on hand for quick preparation in the morning.

YIELD: 2 SERVINGS
PREPARATION TIME: 15 MINUTES
COOKING TIME: 25 MINUTES

INGREDIENTS:
  4 cups vegetable stock, homemade (page 88) or canned
  3 cloves roasted garlic, minced
  1 teaspoon freshly grated ginger
  1-inch piece lemongrass, smashed using the side of a knife
  1-inch length cinnamon stick
  ¼ teaspoon fish sauce
  ¼ teaspoon tamari soy sauce
  ¼ teaspoon red pepper flakes
  ¼ teaspoon sugar
  4 ounces pho rice noodles
  ½ medium tomato, chopped
  1 medium green onion, cut in 1-inch pieces and thinly sliced lengthwise
  ½ cup fresh green soybeans
  1 cup mung bean sprouts, rinsed
  6 sprigs cilantro, leaves only
  1 tablespoon chopped peanuts

1. In a large saucepan, combine stock, garlic, ginger, lemongrass, cinnamon, fish sauce, soy sauce, pepper flakes, and sugar. Bring to a boil, reduce heat, cover, and simmer gently for 20 minutes.
2. Meanwhile, boil four quarts of water in a large saucepan. Remove

from heat, add noodles, and let stand 10 to 15 minutes, until noodles are tender, stirring occasionally. Drain.

3. Strain broth to remove the solid bits. Return broth to pan. Add tomato, green onion, and soybeans to broth. Heat for 5 minutes.

4. Put noodles into serving bowls. Top with mung bean sprouts. Ladle broth and vegetables into the bowls.

5. Top with cilantro and peanuts.

Estimated nutrients per serving:

Calories: 240

Total protein (grams): 9

Soy protein (grams): 6

Total carbohydrate (grams): 40

Total fat (grams): 5

Total fiber (grams): 4

Total fruit and vegetable (servings): 1

For prostate protection:

▪ *To increase lycopene, increase tomato from ½ to 1 medium.*

▪ *For minimal dietary fat, omit peanuts.*

GRIDDLE RICE CAKES

Make sure you have leftover rice on hand to use in these great griddle cakes to accompany Curried Tofu (next recipe).

YIELD: 2 SERVINGS, 2 PANCAKES EACH

PREPARATION TIME: 15 MINUTES

COOKING TIME: 15 MINUTES

INGREDIENTS:

¼ *teaspoon canola oil*

2 *medium green onions, chopped*

1 *cup cooked brown rice (page 178), cold*

1 *cup cooked short grain rice, cold*

1 *tablespoon flour*

1 *small egg, beaten*

⅛ *teaspoon tamari soy sauce*

1. In a medium skillet or wok, heat canola oil over medium-high heat; add green onions and cook, stirring constantly, for 1 minute.
2. In a medium bowl, combine both cups of rice and the green onions, flour, egg, and soy sauce.
3. Form into four patty-shaped cakes.
4. Brush bottom of a nonstick griddle very lightly with oil. Heat over medium heat. Add patties. Cook for 5 minutes on each side.
5. Serve topped with Curried Tofu, below, and accompanied by Fresh Papaya and Mango Chutney, page 120.

Estimated nutrients per serving:
Calories: 260
Total protein (grams): 8
Soy protein (grams): 0
Total carbohydrate (grams): 49
Total fat (grams): 3.5
Total fiber (grams): 3
Total fruit and vegetable (servings): none

For prostate protection: *To eliminate animal products, omit egg and add 1 tablespoon water.*

CURRIED TOFU

For a quick breakfast dish we used commercially available curry powder. The refreshing tastes of fresh lemon juice and cilantro round out the flavors in the dish.

YIELD: 2 SERVINGS
PREPARATION TIME: 10 MINUTES
COOKING TIME: 10 MINUTES

INGREDIENTS:
1 tablespoon cornstarch
¼ teaspoon curry powder
1 cup vegetable stock, homemade (page 88) or canned
½ teaspoon canola oil
¼ small onion, coarsely chopped

¼ *medium green bell pepper, sliced*
¼ *teaspoon freshly squeezed lemon juice*
4 *ounces extra-firm tofu, cubed*
4 *medium cilantro leaves, coarsely chopped*

1. In a small bowl, combine cornstarch and curry powder. Add 2 tablespoons of the stock and stir to make a smooth paste. Add remaining stock. Stir to combine; set aside.
2. In a medium saucepan heat canola oil over medium-high heat. Add onion and green pepper. Cook for 4 minutes or until onion is brown. Add cornstarch mixture and cook, stirring gently and constantly, until mixture comes to a boil and thickens.
3. Add lemon juice and tofu. Stir gently to combine.
4. Spoon over Griddle Rice Cakes, page 51. Top with cilantro leaves. Serve with Fresh Papaya and Mango Chutney, page 120.

Estimated nutrients per serving:
Calories: 60
Total protein (grams): 4
Soy protein (grams): 4
Total carbohydrate (grams): 6
Total fat (grams): 1.5
Total fiber (grams): 1
Total fruit and vegetable (servings): ½

For prostate protection: *For minimal dietary fat, reduce canola oil to ¼ teaspoon.*

MISO SOUP

Having soup for breakfast is a different experience for many people. We find that having this particular soup is soothing and fulfilling. The different textures of the shiitake mushrooms, green onions, and rice are especially appealing. It is a calming way to start the day.

YIELD: 2 SERVINGS
PREPARATION TIME: 15 MINUTES
COOKING TIME: 20 MINUTES

INGREDIENTS:

4 tablespoons miso

4 cups vegetable stock, homemade (page 88) or canned

4 drops chili oil

2 drops sesame oil

¼ teaspoon canola oil

1 medium carrot, thinly sliced on the diagonal

2 medium shiitake mushrooms, sliced

2 medium green onions, quartered lengthwise, then cut into 1½-inch strips

4 ounces extra-firm tofu, slivered

1 cup cooked brown rice (page 178)

1. In a large saucepan, dissolve miso in vegetable stock. Add chili and sesame oils. Bring to a boil.
2. In a medium nonstick skillet, heat canola oil over medium-high heat. Add carrot, mushrooms, and green onions. Cook for 2 minutes. Add to miso-vegetable stock.
3. Return to boiling; reduce heat and simmer for 10 minutes. Add tofu and brown rice. Continue to heat for 2 minutes.

Estimated nutrients per serving:

Calories: 230

Total protein (grams): 12

Soy protein (grams): 8

Total carbohydrate (grams): 38

Total fat (grams): 4.5

Total fiber (grams): 6

Total fruit and vegetable (servings): 1

For prostate protection: You can use this recipe as is.

ENOKI MUSHROOM CUSTARD

These unassuming wispy mushrooms with their long, skinny stems and tiny caps are full of unexpected flavor. Silken tofu used in this recipe adds to the smooth texture of the custard.

YIELD: 2 SERVINGS

PREPARATION TIME: 20 MINUTES

COOKING TIME: 15 MINUTES

INGREDIENTS:

2 ounces silken tofu, sliced

½ teaspoon canola oil

4 medium snow peas, ends and strings removed,
    thinly sliced on the diagonal

2 tablespoons chopped green onion

½ cup 1-inch pieces enoki mushrooms

2 large eggs

⅛ teaspoon tamari soy sauce

⅛ teaspoon freshly grated ginger

½ cup vegetable stock, homemade (page 88) or canned, warm

2 sprinkles cayenne pepper

1. Lightly brush two 8-ounce custard cups or individual casseroles with oil.
2. Place tofu slices on the bottoms of prepared custard dishes.
3. In a medium skillet or wok, heat canola oil over medium-high heat; add snow peas, onion, and mushrooms. Cook for 2 minutes or until soft, stirring constantly. Set aside.
4. In a small bowl, beat the eggs. Add soy sauce, ginger, and stock.
5. Place half of vegetable mixture in each oiled dish. Pour half of the egg mixture over vegetables. Cover with lids or foil.
6. Steam over gently boiling water for 10 minutes or until a knife inserted into the center of the custard comes out clean.
7. Sprinkle with cayenne pepper and serve warm.

Estimated nutrients per serving:

Calories: 110

Total protein (grams): 9

Soy protein (grams): 2

Total carbohydrate (grams): 2

Total fat (grams): 7

Total fiber (grams): 1

Total fruit and vegetable (servings): ½

For prostate protection: *Because this recipe requires egg, it is not suitable for the prostate cancer dietary recommendations.*

CRISPY NOODLES WITH VEGETABLES

Have all the ingredients ready before you start to brown the noodles. Once the noodles are brown and put on the serving dish, quickly stir-fry the vegetables in the same pan.

YIELD: 2 SERVINGS
PREPARATION TIME: 20 MINUTES
COOKING TIME: 20 MINUTES

INGREDIENTS:
   1 (6-ounce) package chuka soba Japanese-style noodles
   1 teaspoon sesame oil
   1½ tablespoons cornstarch
   1 cup water
   2 teaspoons hoisin sauce
   1 teaspoon tamari soy sauce
   1 teaspoon canola oil
   ¼ cup chopped green onion
   1 small carrot, thinly sliced on the diagonal
   1 cup fresh green soybeans
   8 ears baby corn, cut into 1-inch lengths

1. Cook noodles according to package directions. Drain; do not rinse.
2. Put noodles in a medium bowl. Add sesame oil; stir to mix. Set aside while you prepare the vegetables.
3. In a small bowl, combine cornstarch with ¼ cup of the water to make a smooth paste. Add remaining water, hoisin sauce, and soy sauce. Stir to combine; set aside.
4. In a large skillet or wok, heat the canola oil over high heat. Add noodles; cook until noodles start to get brown, tossing constantly with chopsticks or tongs. Transfer to two serving dishes.
5. Reduce heat to medium. Immediately add green onion, carrot, soybeans, and corn to the skillet. Cook for 2 minutes.
6. Add cornstarch mixture; stir constantly until sauce comes to a boil, about 1 minute.
7. To serve, spoon vegetable mixture over noodles.

Estimated nutrients per serving:
Calories: 430
Total protein (grams): 15
Soy protein (grams): 11
Total carbohydrate (grams): 71
Total fat (grams): 11
Total fiber (grams): 6
Total fruit and vegetable (servings): 1

For prostate protection:
■ *To increase lycopene, add 1 medium tomato, chopped, with the other vegetables in step 5.*
■ *For minimal dietary fat, reduce canola oil to ½ teaspoon.*

GRILLED MARINATED MUSHROOMS AND TOMATOES

For breakfast dishes, mushrooms and tomatoes are surprisingly good flavors when combined. This combination is enhanced by the different intensities of the crimini and button mushrooms. Don't be alarmed by the tablespoon of oil used in the marinade — most of it drips off during cooking.

YIELD: 2 SERVINGS
PREPARATION TIME: 10 MINUTES
COOKING TIME: 5 MINUTES

INGREDIENTS:
1 tablespoon sesame oil
1 tablespoon tamari soy sauce
1 teaspoon rice vinegar
2 drops chili oil
½ teaspoon honey
4 medium button mushrooms, stems trimmed
4 medium crimini (brown) mushrooms, stems trimmed
8 large cherry tomatoes
2 cups cooked brown rice (page 178)

Preheat broiler.

1. In a small teacup or bowl, combine sesame oil, soy sauce, vinegar, chili oil, and honey.
2. Thread mushrooms and tomatoes alternately on skewers. Brush with soy sauce mixture.
3. Place skewers on a broiler pan. Place pan under preheated broiler for 2 minutes.
4. Brush again with mixture. Turn over; broil for 2 more minutes.
5. Serve over rice.

Estimated nutrients per serving:

Calories: 250
Total protein (grams): 7
Soy protein (grams): 0
Total carbohydrate (grams): 51
Total fat (grams): 2
Total fiber (grams): 5
Total fruit and vegetable (servings): 1

For prostate protection: *For minimal dietary fat, use marinade sparingly.*

EGG FOO YUNG

In China the egg is a symbol of good luck. In this traditional Chinese egg dish, a mixture of vegetables and eggs is formed into "pancakes" and grilled quickly. It provides the basis for a nice breakfast.

YIELD: 2 SERVINGS, 2 PANCAKES EACH
PREPARATION TIME: 15 MINUTES
COOKING TIME: 10 MINUTES

INGREDIENTS:

½ tablespoon cornstarch
1 tablespoon water
⅓ cup vegetable stock, homemade (page 88) or canned
1 teaspoon tamari soy sauce
¼ teaspoon seasoned rice vinegar
¼ teaspoon canola oil

1 *small green onion, chopped*
2 *small button mushrooms, chopped*
¼ *cup bean sprouts*
2 *ounces silken tofu*
2 *large eggs*
1 *large egg white*

1. In a small saucepan, combine cornstarch and water to make a smooth paste. Add stock, soy sauce, and vinegar. Stir to combine. Cook over medium-high heat, stirring gently and constantly, until mixture comes to a full boil. Cover, remove from heat, and set aside.
2. In a medium skillet or wok, heat the canola oil over medium heat; add green onion and mushrooms. Cook for 2 minutes or until mushrooms are soft, stirring constantly. Add bean sprouts and remove from heat.
3. In a medium bowl, beat tofu with a fork. Add eggs and egg white. Continue beating with fork. Add vegetables.
4. Brush bottom of a nonstick griddle very lightly with oil. Heat over medium-high heat. Add ¼ cup of the egg mixture for each pancake. Cook until the egg is set, about 1 minute. Turn over and cook until the underside is golden.
5. Serve topped with sauce.

Estimated nutrients per serving:
Calories: 110
Total protein (grams): 10
Soy protein (grams): 2
Total carbohydrate (grams): 4
Total fat (grams): 6
Total fiber (grams): 0.5
Total fruit and vegetable (servings): ½

For prostate protection: *Because this recipe requires egg, it is not suitable for the prostate cancer dietary recommendations.*

RICE WRAPS

Although our menu plan calls for these easy-to-make rice wraps to accompany Egg Foo Yung, they are also great with other dishes or on their own as a snack. The filling got especially high marks from one of the taste judges. She loved the crystallized ginger.

YIELD: 2 SERVINGS
PREPARATION TIME: 15 MINUTES
COOKING TIME: 5 MINUTES

INGREDIENTS:
1 large green onion
½ teaspoon canola oil
¼ medium red pepper, cut into thin strips about 1 inch long
1 teaspoon finely chopped crystallized ginger
6 slices water chestnuts, chopped
1 cup hot cooked rice
½ teaspoon sesame oil
4 drops chili oil
4 spring roll wrappers

1. Slice the green part of the green onion into thin slices. Cut the white part in long, thin strips, about 1½ inches long.
2. In a medium skillet or wok, heat the canola oil over medium-high heat; add red pepper, green onion, ginger, and water chestnuts. Cook for 2 minutes, stirring constantly.
3. In a medium bowl, combine the rice with the vegetable mixture. Add sesame and chili oils. Stir gently to combine.
4. Soften spring roll wrappers in water. When soft, put one wrapper on a flat surface covered with a paper towel. Blot the top side of the wrapper with another paper towel. Place one-fourth of the rice mixture on one end of the wrapper to form a "log." Fold the sides of the wrapper toward the middle, then roll tightly to enclose the filling.

Estimated nutrients per serving:
Calories: 210
Total protein (grams): 5
Soy protein (grams): 0
Total carbohydrate (grams): 41
Total fat (grams): 3.5
Total fiber (grams): 3
Total fruit and vegetable (servings): ½

For prostate protection: *For minimal dietary fat, reduce canola oil to ¼ teaspoon.*

ASPARAGUS AND CARROT IN OYSTER SAUCE

The vibrant, contrasting colors and flavors of the carrot and asparagus are pleasing to the eyes as well as to the palate.

YIELD: 2 SERVINGS

PREPARATION TIME: 10 MINUTES

COOKING TIME: 10 MINUTES

INGREDIENTS:

½ tablespoon cornstarch
½ cup vegetable stock, homemade (page 88) or canned
1 teaspoon oyster sauce
¼ teaspoon honey
¼ teaspoon rice vinegar
6 drops chili oil
4 ounces Asian-style vermicelli noodles
½ teaspoon canola oil
1 small carrot, sliced on the diagonal
8 spears asparagus, tough ends trimmed, sliced on the diagonal

1. In a small bowl, combine cornstarch with 2 tablespoons of the vegetable stock to make a smooth paste. Add remaining stock, oyster sauce, honey, vinegar, and chili oil. Stir to combine; set aside.
2. Cook noodles according to package directions. Drain; keep warm.
3. In a medium skillet or wok, heat canola oil over medium-high heat; add carrot. Cook for 2 minutes, stirring constantly. Add asparagus; cook for 2 more minutes.
4. Add cornstarch mixture; stir constantly until sauce comes to a boil.
5. Serve over noodles.

Estimated nutrients per serving:
Calories: 180
Total protein (grams): 4

Soy protein (grams): 0
Total carbohydrate (grams): 37
Total fat (grams): 1.5
Total fiber (grams): 2
Total fruit and vegetable (servings): 1

For prostate protection: *For minimal dietary fat, reduce canola oil to ¼ teaspoon.*

NEW AMERICAN

HOMEMADE MUESLI

This cereal is a favorite of the Swiss. The whole grains are uncooked, so the taste may be unfamiliar initially. However, it will soon be a favorite, because it is as easy to prepare as it is good to eat. Because muesli stores well, we also give ingredient quantities for 16 servings. Store the combined dry ingredients in an airtight container in a cool, dry place for a quick and easy workday breakfast.

YIELD: 2 SERVINGS, ½ CUP EACH (AMOUNTS ARE
ALSO GIVEN FOR 16 SERVINGS TO MAKE AHEAD)
PREPARATION TIME: 10 MINUTES
COOKING TIME: NONE

INGREDIENTS (QUANTITIES FOR 16 SERVINGS ARE
IN PARENTHESES):
½ cup (4 cups) rolled oats
¼ cup (2 cups) wheat flakes
2 tablespoons (1 cup) packed soy protein powder
1 tablespoon (½ cup) oat bran
1 tablespoon (½ cup) slivered almonds, toasted
4 halves (32 halves) dried apricots, chopped
¼ cup nonfat soy milk
¼ cup plain nonfat yogurt

1. Combine all dry ingredients.
2. Serve ½ cup in each bowl.
3. Add soy milk.
4. Top with yogurt.

Estimated nutrients per serving:
Calories: 230
Total protein (grams): 17
Soy protein (grams): 9

Total carbohydrate (grams): 35
Total fat (grams): 4.5
Total fiber (grams): 5
Total fruit and vegetable (servings): ½

For prostate protection:
- *For minimal dietary fat, omit almonds.*
- *To eliminate animal products, omit nonfat yogurt.*

STEEL-CUT OATMEAL WITH SUN-DRIED CRANBERRIES AND WALNUTS

Steel-cut oats contain the entire oat kernel, including the oat bran and germ. The coarse texture and high fiber content of steel-cut oats increase the time needed for cooking. This variety of oatmeal is commonly used in the British Isles and is available in most supermarkets in the United States. For a quick preparation in the morning, soak oatmeal in the water overnight. In the morning, bring to a boil, reduce heat, and simmer for 10 minutes.

YIELD: 2 SERVINGS
PREPARATION TIME: 5 MINUTES
COOKING TIME: 25 MINUTES

INGREDIENTS:
    2 cups water
    ½ cup steel-cut oats
    Pinch salt
    2 tablespoons packed soy protein powder
    ¼ cup nonfat dry milk powder
    2 teaspoons toasted wheat germ
    1 tablespoon dried cranberries
    2 teaspoons chopped walnuts
    ¼ cup nonfat soy milk

1. Bring water to a rolling boil in a heavy saucepan.
2. Add oats and salt and stir immediately. Reduce heat to low and cook for 20 to 25 minutes, until of desired thickness. Stir frequently to avoid sticking. Do not allow oats to boil over.

3. Stir in soy protein powder and milk powder.
4. Pour into 2 bowls. Top with wheat germ, cranberries, walnuts, and soy milk.

Estimated nutrients per serving:
Calories: 200
Total protein (grams): 16
Soy protein (grams): 9
Total carbohydrate (grams): 27
Total fat (grams): 7
Total fiber (grams): 4
Total fruit and vegetable (servings): ½

For prostate protection:
- *For minimal dietary fat, omit walnuts.*
- *To eliminate animal products, omit nonfat milk powder.*

EGGS FLORENTINE

This makes a nice entrée for a leisurely weekend brunch. This dish is an excellent source of many nutrients; the spinach is an outstanding source of beta-carotene, folic acid, and vitamin C.

YIELD: 2 SERVINGS
PREPARATION TIME: 15 MINUTES
COOKING TIME: 20 TO 25 MINUTES

INGREDIENTS:
4 cups packed fresh spinach leaves
½ cup basic white sauce (page 90)
1 tablespoon freshly grated Parmesan cheese
2 large eggs

Preheat oven to 350 degrees.
1. Wash spinach thoroughly; chop coarsely. Put in a heavy saucepan with only the water clinging to the leaves. Bring to a boil, cover, reduce heat, and cook for 3 minutes.
2. Drain spinach, combine with white sauce and Parmesan cheese.

3. Divide between 2 individual ovenproof dishes (about 5 inches in diameter). Make a well in the center of spinach mixture in each dish. Gently crack one egg into each well.
4. Cover with foil, place in preheated oven.
5. Bake for 20 minutes, until egg white is set and yolk is soft. Bake an additional 5 minutes if a hard yolk is desired.

Estimated nutrients per serving:
Calories: 130
Total protein (grams): 11
Soy protein (grams): 0
Total carbohydrate (grams): 8
Total fat (grams): 6
Total fiber (grams): 2
Total fruit and vegetable (servings): 2

For prostate protection: *To eliminate animal products, use 4 ounces of baked tofu in place of the eggs and make the basic white sauce with nonfat soy milk instead of nonfat milk; sprinkle with toasted whole wheat bread crumbs as garnish instead of baking with Parmesan cheese.*

BUCKWHEAT PANCAKES WITH BERRIES

Buckwheat is not really wheat at all. It is the seed of a low-growing bush native to Siberia. Barbara especially enjoys the combination of the sweet, tangy berries with the nutty flavor of the buckwheat. Frozen berries that have been thawed can be substituted for fresh ones.

YIELD: 2 SERVINGS, 4 SMALL PANCAKES EACH
PREPARATION TIME: 15 MINUTES, PLUS 30
     MINUTES' STANDING TIME
COOKING TIME: 15 MINUTES

INGREDIENTS:
⅓ cup buckwheat flour
⅓ cup whole wheat flour
½ teaspoon baking powder
Pinch salt

2 tablespoons packed soy protein powder
1 large egg, separated
1 cup nonfat soy milk
⅛ teaspoon canola oil
1 cup fresh berries

1. Mix flours, baking powder, salt, and soy protein powder in a medium bowl.
2. In a small bowl, stir together the egg yolk and soy milk until well blended.
3. Add egg mixture to dry ingredients; stir again until the mixture is well blended.
4. Cover; let stand 30 minutes.
5. In a small bowl, beat egg whites until soft peaks form when the beaters are lifted. Gently fold egg whites into batter.
6. Heat nonstick skillet over medium heat. Wipe a tiny amount of canola oil over the bottom of the skillet.
7. Pour ¼ cup of batter for each pancake onto skillet. Cook until a few bubbles appear in batter. Turn over, cook 1 to 2 minutes longer, until lightly browned.
8. Put 4 pancakes on each plate; add berries.

Estimated nutrients per serving:
Calories: 280
Total protein (grams): 20
Soy protein (grams): 11
Total carbohydrate (grams): 44
Total fat (grams): 4.5
Total fiber (grams): 7
Total fruit and vegetable (servings): 1

For prostate protection: *To eliminate animal products, omit egg and increase nonfat soy milk to 1 cup plus 2 tablespoons; increase baking powder to ¾ tablespoon.*

CRUNCHY HOMEMADE GRANOLA

Every household needs a basic granola recipe. We developed this granola for friends who wanted a simple recipe they could prepare quickly. A handful of our granola late in the afternoon is a great pick-me-up and will hold you until dinner. This recipe is very easy to prepare, which is a real plus.

YIELD: 4 SERVINGS
PREPARATION TIME: 10 MINUTES
COOKING TIME: 45 MINUTES

INGREDIENTS:

2 cups rolled oats
¼ cup packed soy protein powder
¼ cup nonfat dry milk powder
2 tablespoons sliced almonds
½ cup apple juice concentrate
2 tablespoons brown sugar
1 teaspoon canola oil
⅛ teaspoon salt
1 tablespoon chopped dried apricots
1 tablespoon raisins
1¼ cups nonfat soy milk

Preheat oven to 250 degrees.

1. In a large bowl, combine oats, soy protein powder, milk powder, and almonds.
2. In a small bowl, mix apple juice concentrate, brown sugar, oil, and salt.
3. Add juice mixture to oat mix; stir until evenly moistened.
4. Spread on a cookie sheet. Bake in preheated oven for 45 minutes, stirring every 15 minutes to prevent burning.
5. Mix in apricots and raisins.
6. Pour soy milk over cereal.

Estimated nutrients per serving:

Calories: 370
Total protein (grams): 19
Soy protein (grams): 10
Total carbohydrate (grams): 62
Total fat (grams): 7
Total fiber (grams): 6
Total fruit and vegetable (servings): 1

For prostate protection:
  ■ *To eliminate animal products, omit nonfat dry milk powder.*
  ■ *For minimal dietary fat, omit almonds.*

SUPER TOAST WITH GINGER YOGURT

This is a modification of a recipe that Rita's children named "super toast" because they liked it so much. It was always the breakfast they requested for birthdays and other special occasions, and Rita was happy to comply with their request because it is so easy to prepare.

YIELD: 2 SERVINGS

PREPARATION TIME: 15 MINUTES

COOKING TIME: NONE

INGREDIENTS:

1 large Fuji apple
¼ cup apple juice
½ teaspoon chopped crystallized ginger
2 slices French bread, sliced ½ to ¾ inch thick
¼ cup plain nonfat yogurt
½ teaspoon powdered ginger
1 medium dried black mission fig, sliced

1. Core and slice apple; put in a small saucepan with apple juice and crystallized ginger.
2. Bring slowly to a boil, turn down heat, and cook gently for 10 minutes or until soft.
3. Drain apple; reserve crystallized ginger and 1 tablespoon of juice.
4. Toast bread.
5. Meanwhile, mix yogurt, powdered ginger, and reserved crystallized ginger and juice in a small bowl.
6. Place one slice of toast on each of 2 plates.
7. Arrange apple slices on top of toast, top with yogurt mixture, and decorate with sliced fig.

Estimated nutrients per serving:
Calories: 220
Total protein (grams): 5

Soy protein (grams): 0
Total carbohydrate (grams): 47
Total fat (grams): 2
Total fiber (grams): 5
Total fruit and vegetable (servings): 1

For prostate protection: *To eliminate animal products, substitute silken tofu for the nonfat yogurt in the topping.*

DATE-ORANGE MUFFINS

Don't be surprised when these muffins don't rise as you would expect. The wheat bran and whole wheat flours inhibit the rising. In this recipe, a deep brown color is not an indication that the muffin is done. The soy protein powder causes them to be browner than usual. Continue to bake until a toothpick inserted in the center comes out clean.

YIELD: 5 SERVINGS, 2 MUFFINS PER SERVING
PREPARATION TIME: 20 MINUTES
COOKING TIME: 40 TO 45 MINUTES

INGREDIENTS:
 ½ cup chopped dates
 ¼ cup wheat bran
 ½ cup orange juice concentrate
 ¾ cup hot water
 1 large egg, beaten
 ¼ cup light brown sugar
 1 tablespoon extra-light olive oil
 1 cup whole wheat flour
 ½ cup all-purpose flour
 2 tablespoons packed soy protein powder
 1½ teaspoons baking powder

Preheat oven to 350 degrees.
1. In a medium bowl combine dates and bran. Add orange juice concentrate and hot water; let soak for 15 minutes.
2. In another bowl combine egg and brown sugar. Add olive oil and beat until well mixed.

3. In a third bowl, combine flours, soy protein powder, and baking powder.
4. Stir date-orange mixture into egg mixture.
5. Gently combine egg and flour mixtures. Do not beat.
6. Pour batter into 10 nonstick muffin cups that have been brushed with extra-light olive oil.
7. Bake in preheated oven for 40 to 45 minutes or until a toothpick inserted in the center of a muffin comes out clean.
8. Let cool in the pan for 5 to 10 minutes before removing muffins.

Estimated nutrients per serving:
Calories: 310
Total protein (grams): 11
Soy protein (grams): 3
Total carbohydrate (grams): 64
Total fat (grams): 5
Total fiber (grams): 6
Total fruit and vegetable (servings): 1

For prostate protection: *This recipe cannot be modified to meet the prostate cancer recommendations.*

RYE BAGEL WITH SAVORY SPREAD

Make this spread ahead of time to let the flavors develop. The recipe can be doubled to have on hand for a quick breakfast later; it keeps well in the refrigerator for as long as a week.

YIELD: 2 SERVINGS
PREPARATION TIME: 10 MINUTES
COOKING TIME: NONE

INGREDIENTS:
1 tablespoon packed soy protein powder
¼ cup Neufchâtel cheese (reduced-fat cream cheese)
4 teaspoons nonfat soy milk
Pinch salt
½ teaspoon basil

1 teaspoon chopped fresh chives
2 large cloves roasted garlic, crushed
2 large rye bagels

1. Blend soy protein powder into Neufchâtel. Gradually stir in soy milk.
2. Stir in salt, basil, chives, and garlic.
3. Toast the bagels if you wish. Spread with soy mixture.

Estimated nutrients per serving:
  Calories: 310
  Total protein (grams): 11
  Soy protein (grams): 4
  Total carbohydrate (grams): 46
  Total fat (grams): 8
  Total fiber (grams): 4
  Total fruit and vegetable (servings): none

For prostate protection: *This recipe cannot be modified to meet the prostate cancer recommendations.*

COFFEE CAKE

This is an adaptation of a popular family recipe. The taste is excellent. The whole wheat makes each bite satisfying. The mild cinnamon-apple taste is especially appealing. The coffee cake is wonderful for breakfast but also as an afternoon snack.

YIELD: 6 SERVINGS
PREPARATION TIME: 20 MINUTES
COOKING TIME: 35 MINUTES

INGREDIENTS:
  ½ cup soy flour
  1½ cups whole wheat flour
  1 teaspoon baking powder
  1 teaspoon baking soda
  ⅛ teaspoon salt

⅛ *teaspoon cinnamon*
1 *large egg*
1 *cup brown sugar*
2 *tablespoons applesauce*
¼ *cup extra-light olive oil*
¼ *cup nonfat buttermilk*
½ *large Fuji apple, grated, not peeled*

Preheat oven to 350 degrees.

1. Stir together flours, baking powder, baking soda, salt, and cinnamon.
2. In another bowl, beat egg. Mix in brown sugar and applesauce.
3. Add olive oil to the egg mixture and beat until well blended. Stir in buttermilk. Add grated apple.
4. Make a well in the center of flour mixture. Pour in egg mixture; stir gently until just mixed. Do not beat.
5. Pour batter into a nonstick 8×8-inch pan that has been lightly brushed with extra-light olive oil.
6. Bake in preheated oven for 35 minutes or until a toothpick inserted into the center comes out clean.

Estimated nutrients per serving:
Calories: 340
Total protein (grams): 9
Soy protein (grams): 4
Total carbohydrate (grams): 65
Total fat (grams): 11
Total fiber (grams): 6
Total fruit and vegetable (servings): none

For prostate protection: *This recipe cannot be modified to meet the prostate cancer recommendations.*

MEDITERRANEAN

GOAT CHEESE WITH MELON AND FIGS

The tastes and textures of the fresh fruits are a great contrast with the tangy goat cheese. Even when time is short, you can have this special breakfast.

YIELD: 2 SERVINGS
PREPARATION TIME: 10 MINUTES
COOKING TIME: NONE

INGREDIENTS:
  2 ounces reduced-fat goat cheese, sliced
  4 medium fresh figs, sliced
  ½ medium casaba melon, peeled and sliced

Arrange the cheese and fruits on 2 individual serving plates.

Estimated nutrients per serving:
  Calories: 240
  Total protein (grams): 8
  Soy protein (grams): 0
  Total carbohydrate (grams): 35
  Total fat (grams): 9
  Total fiber (grams): 4
  Total fruit and vegetable (servings): 2

For prostate protection: For minimal dietary fat, use 1 ounce of goat cheese and a whole casaba melon.

ARTICHOKE FRITTATA

This tastes great hot from the oven or at room temperature. If you prepare it ahead, refrigerate, then bring to room temperature before serving. Leftovers travel well and make a nice lunch.

YIELD: 4 SERVINGS
PREPARATION TIME: 20 MINUTES
COOKING TIME: 35 MINUTES

INGREDIENTS:

1 tablespoon olive oil
½ medium sweet red pepper, stems, seeds,
  and membranes removed; sliced
½ medium green bell pepper, stems, seeds,
  and membranes removed; sliced
2 medium green onions, sliced
1 clove roasted garlic, minced
1¾ ounces savory baked tofu, cut in ¼-inch dice
1 cup canned artichoke hearts, quartered
2 tablespoons chopped parsley
½ teaspoon oregano
½ teaspoon salt
⅛ teaspoon pepper
2 large eggs
4 large egg whites
¼ cup nonfat milk
1 tablespoon freshly grated Parmesan cheese

Preheat oven to 350 degrees.

1. In a large overnproof, nonstick skillet, heat olive oil over medium heat. Add red and green peppers, onions, and garlic. Cook for 5 minutes.
2. Add tofu, artichoke hearts, parsley, oregano, salt, and pepper. Mix gently. Reduce heat to very low.
3. In a small bowl, combine eggs, egg whites, and milk. Beat with a fork until well blended but not frothy.
4. Distribute eggs evenly over vegetables. Do not stir.
5. Cook, uncovered, over very low heat for about 15 minutes.
6. Put in preheated oven for 5 to 8 minutes until top is set but not brown.
7. Remove from oven. Sprinkle with Parmesan cheese and let sit for 5 minutes.

Estimated nutrients per serving:
Calories: 170
Total protein (grams): 11

Soy protein (grams): 1
Total carbohydrate (grams): 17
Total fat (grams): 7
Total fiber (grams): 5
Total fruit and vegetable (servings): 2

For prostate protection: *You can use this recipe as is.*

CORNMEAL WAFFLES WITH PEACHES AND BERRIES

The cornmeal imparts a delightful crunchy texture to these waffles. The soy protein powder and soy milk provide a good amount of soy protein. The waffles are especially good in the summer when fresh peaches and berries are available. However, frozen or canned berries and peaches also work well.

YIELD: 2 SERVINGS
PREPARATION TIME: 20 MINUTES
COOKING TIME: 20 MINUTES

INGREDIENTS:
1 large peach, sliced
1 cup blueberries
½ cup whole wheat flour
¼ cup cornmeal
2 tablespoons packed soy protein powder
Pinch salt
2 teaspoons baking powder
1 tablespoon brown sugar
1 large egg, separated
1 cup nonfat soy milk

Preheat waffle iron according to manufacturer's instructions.
1. Combine peach and blueberries in a small bowl. Set aside.
2. Stir together flour, cornmeal, soy protein powder, salt, baking powder, and brown sugar in a medium bowl.
3. In a small bowl, beat egg yolk; add soy milk and mix until blended.

4. In another bowl, beat egg white until it forms soft peaks when the blade is lifted.
5. Make a well in the dry ingredients; pour egg and soy mixture into the flour mixture. Stir gently to combine.
6. Gently fold in the beaten egg whites. Do not beat.
7. Bake in preheated waffle iron according to manufacturer's directions.
8. Top with fruit.

Estimated nutrients per serving:
Calories: 410
Total protein (grams): 21
Soy protein (grams): 11
Total carbohydrate (grams): 73
Total fat (grams): 4.5
Total fiber (grams): 9
Total fruit and vegetable (servings): 2

For prostate protection: *You can use this recipe as is.*

BUCKWHEAT CREPES WITH DATE-ORANGE FILLING

Dates and oranges, two fruits of the Mediterranean region, combine to make a tasty filling that contrasts with the nutty flavor of the buckwheat and the tangy flavor of the yogurt.

YIELD: 2 SERVINGS, 2 CREPES EACH
PREPARATION TIME: 10 MINUTES, PLUS 1 HOUR'S
   STANDING TIME
COOKING TIME: 20 MINUTES

INGREDIENTS
2 tablespoons buckwheat flour
2 tablespoons whole wheat flour
1 large egg
3 tablespoons nonfat milk
2 tablespoons orange juice
2 medium oranges, peeled and chopped

2 medium dates, pitted and chopped
6 tablespoons plain nonfat yogurt
¼ cup orange juice

1. Stir together buckwheat and whole wheat flours in medium bowl.
2. In a small bowl, combine egg, milk, and the 2 tablespoons of orange juice.
3. Make a well in flour mixture; add milk mixture and stir to combine. Refrigerate for 1 hour.
4. Combine oranges and dates for the filling.
5. Stir together yogurt and the ¼ cup orange juice until smooth for the topping.
6. Heat an 8-inch nonstick skillet over medium heat. Wipe with a tiny amount of canola oil over the bottom of the skillet.
7. Pour a small amount of batter (a little less than ¼ cup) into the skillet. Quickly swirl the skillet around to distribute the batter evenly in a thin layer over the bottom of the skillet. Cook for 2 minutes, until lightly browned.
8. Turn over with a spatula and cook for 2 minutes on the other side.
9. Transfer to a serving plate. Put one-fourth of the filling mixture in a line on the center of each crepe; roll up.
10. Serve 2 crepes, seam down, on each plate. Drizzle with yogurt topping.

Estimated nutrients per serving:
   Calories: 240
   Total protein (grams): 10
   Soy protein (grams): 0
   Total carbohydrate (grams): 42
   Total fat (grams): 4.5
   Total fiber (grams): 6
   Total fruit and vegetable (servings): 1

For prostate protection: *You can use this recipe as is.*

PEACH-ORANGE SMOOTHIE

The texture of this smoothie depends on the peach slices' and orange juice concentrate's being frozen. Slice the peach and freeze overnight.

Frozen peaches are always available and can be used when fresh peaches are out of season.

YIELD: 2 SERVINGS
PREPARATION TIME: 5 MINUTES
COOKING TIME: NONE

INGREDIENTS:
   ½ cup plain nonfat yogurt
   1½ cups vanilla nonfat soy milk
   1 medium peach, sliced and frozen
   ½ cup frozen orange juice concentrate
   Pinch nutmeg

1. Combine all ingredients except nutmeg in a blender.
2. Blend for 30 seconds.
3. Pour into 2 glasses. Sprinkle with nutmeg.

Estimated nutrients per serving:
   Calories: 250
   Total protein (grams): 10
   Soy protein (grams): 5
   Total carbohydrate (grams): 47
   Total fat (grams): 0.5
   Total fiber (grams): 3
   Total fruit and vegetable (servings): 2

For prostate protection: *You can use this recipe as is.*

SAVORY BREAKFAST ROLL

Occasionally Barbara would show up at a cooking session with a bag of ingredients and a special grin on her face and say, "I have a great idea!" This idea produced a really great recipe. For a book group we belong to, we tried a slight variation that can work as an appetizer. We spread the ricotta mixture on thin baguette slices, topped them with the sweet red pepper slices, sprinkled them with fresh parsley and Parmesan cheese, then popped them into the oven for a few minutes.

The ricotta and tofu mixture makes a creamy filling, and the red pepper adds a great crunch. They got rave reviews!

YIELD: 2 SERVINGS

PREPARATION TIME: 15 MINUTES

COOKING TIME: 6 MINUTES

INGREDIENTS:

1 baguette

¼ cup low-fat ricotta cheese

¼ cup silken tofu

2 tablespoons packed soy protein powder

1 tablespoon sliced black olives

¼ teaspoon oregano

1 tablespoon chopped Italian parsley

¼ medium sweet red pepper, stems, seeds,
    and membranes removed; sliced

1 teaspoon freshly grated Parmesan cheese

Preheat oven to 350 degrees.

1. Cut baguette in half lengthwise but do not separate. Place in oven 3 minutes.
2. In a small bowl, combine ricotta cheese, tofu, and soy protein powder. Mix well. Stir in olives, oregano, and half of the parsley.
3. Separate roll into two halves. Remove some of the dough from the center of each half to make a well. Place roll halves crust down on a cookie sheet.
4. Put half of the ricotta mixture into each roll. Spread evenly to within ½ inch of the edge of the roll.
5. Top with pepper slices. Return to oven and bake, uncovered, for three minutes
6. Sprinkle with Parmesan cheese and remaining parsley.

Estimated nutrients per serving:

Calories: 350

Total protein (grams): 19

Soy protein (grams): 10

Total carbohydrate (grams): 59

Total fat (grams): 6

Total fiber (grams): 5
Total fruit and vegetable (servings): none

For prostate protection: *You can use this recipe as is.*

COUSCOUS WITH DRIED FRUIT AND ALMONDS

Couscous is a form of tiny pasta commonly used in countries of the Mediterranean region. It is easy and quick to prepare, so using the instant variety is unnecessary. Prepare the fruits and almonds ahead of time and store in an airtight container to hasten morning preparation time.

YIELD: 2 SERVINGS
PREPARATION TIME: 10 MINUTES
COOKING TIME: NONE

INGREDIENTS:
½ cup couscous
¾ cup boiling water
2 medium dates, pitted and chopped
2 medium dried figs, chopped
2 halves dried apricots, chopped
1 tablespoon slivered almonds, toasted
½ cup plain nonfat yogurt
½ cup orange juice

1. Put couscous in a medium bowl. Pour the boiling water over couscous. Let stand 5 minutes.
2. Fluff couscous with a fork. Mix in fruits and almonds.
3. Divide between two bowls. Combine yogurt and orange juice, spoon over the top of couscous.

Estimated nutrients per serving:
Calories: 330
Total protein (grams): 11
Soy protein (grams): 0

Total carbohydrate (grams): 66
Total fat (grams): 3
Total fiber (grams): 5
Total fruit and vegetable (servings): 1

For prostate protection: *You can use this recipe as is.*

DATE BREAKFAST BARS

Rita's daughter Laura likes to take a couple of batches of these bars back to college with her after she's been home on break. Her friends all look forward to having them as study break snacks. The bars travel well in a sealed plastic bag. Bake the bars on the weekend to have for breakfast or a snack during the week. One taste judge commented, "This is absolutely delicious. It's crunchy and yet moist, and the contrasting texture of the dates and walnuts is very satisfying. It's very sweet, which I love. I would even serve this as a dessert!"

YIELD: 8 SERVINGS
PREPARATION TIME: 15 MINUTES
COOKING TIME: 35 MINUTES

INGREDIENTS:
 ½ *cup whole wheat flour*
 2 *tablespoons packed soy protein powder*
 1 *teaspoon baking powder*
 1¼ *teaspoons cinnamon*
 1½ *cups rolled oats*
 ½ *cup chopped pitted dates*
 ¼ *cup chopped walnuts*
 1 *large egg*
 ½ *cup brown sugar*
 ¼ *cup white sugar*
 ¼ *cup extra-light olive oil*
 ½ *cup applesauce*
 ⅛ *teaspoon vanilla extract*

Preheat oven to 350 degrees.

1. Stir together flour, protein powder, baking powder, and cinnamon. Add oats, dates, and walnuts and stir to combine.
2. In another bowl, beat egg. Add sugars and beat until well blended. Add olive oil; continue beating until well mixed. Stir in applesauce and vanilla.
3. Make a well in the center of flour mixture. Pour in egg mixture, stir gently until just mixed. Do not beat.
4. Spread mixture in an 8×8-inch nonstick pan that has been lightly brushed with olive oil. Bake in preheated oven for 35 minutes or until toothpick inserted in the center comes out clean.
5. Remove from oven and cool for 10 minutes before removing from pan.

Estimated nutrients per serving:
Calories: 300
Total protein (grams): 7
Soy protein (grams): 2
Total carbohydrate (grams): 46
Total fat (grams): 12
Total fiber (grams): 4
Total fruit and vegetable (servings): none

For prostate protection: *You can use this recipe as is.*

GRILLED GRAPEFRUIT HALF

Grilled grapefruit halves are an elegant addition to any breakfast. They are so simple and quick to prepare that you can serve them often. The sweetened, warm, grilled grapefruit is a good addition to a breakfast in winter, when you might not want a cold grapefruit first thing in the morning.

YIELD: 2 SERVINGS
PREPARATION TIME: 10 MINUTES
COOKING TIME: 5 MINUTES

INGREDIENTS:

1 medium grapefruit
2 teaspoons brown sugar
1 large strawberry, cut in half lengthwise

Preheat broiler.
1. Cut the grapefruit in half. Cut around each segment with a serrated knife.
2. Sprinkle with brown sugar.
3. Place grapefruit halves on baking sheet.
4. Place under preheated broiler for 3 to 5 minutes, until brown sugar melts.
5. Top with strawberry, flat side down.

Estimated nutrients per serving:
Calories: 60
Total protein (grams): 1
Soy protein (grams): 0
Total carbohydrate (grams): 15
Total fat (grams): 0
Total fiber (grams): 2
Total fruit and vegetable (servings): 1

For prostate protection: *You can use this recipe as is.*

OLIVE SODA BREAD

The Irish claim to have originated soda bread, which is now enjoyed throughout the world. We took artistic license and created a soda bread using flavors of the Mediterranean region. The rising agent in soda bread is baking soda, which starts to act as soon as it gets wet. So have the pan ready and work quickly after you combine the liquid and the flour mixture. Like all quick breads, it is best served soon after it comes out of the oven because it does not retain its moisture.

YIELD: 8 SERVINGS

PREPARATION TIME: 20 MINUTES

COOKING TIME: 40 MINUTES

INGREDIENTS:

1 cup whole wheat flour
½ cup all-purpose flour
½ cup soy flour
¼ teaspoon salt
1½ teaspoons baking powder
½ teaspoon baking soda
1 large egg, beaten
1 tablespoon extra-virgin olive oil
1 cup nonfat buttermilk
2 tablespoons sliced olives

Preheat oven to 375 degrees.

1. In a large bowl, combine flours, salt, baking powder, and baking soda.
2. In another bowl, combine beaten egg and olive oil. Stir in buttermilk and olives.
3. Make a well in the center of flour mixture. Pour in egg mixture; stir gently until just mixed. Do not beat.
4. Spread batter in a nonstick 8-inch round pan that has been brushed lightly with olive oil.
5. Bake in preheated oven for 40 minutes or until toothpick inserted in the center comes out clean.

Estimated nutrients per serving:

Calories: 140
Total protein (grams): 8
Soy protein (grams): 3
Total carbohydrate (grams): 21
Total fat (grams): 3
Total fiber (grams): 3
Total fruit and vegetable (servings): none

For prostate protection: *You can use this recipe as is.*

CITRUS DELIGHT

This recipe is best prepared the night before because longer soaking allows the prunes to get really plump.

YIELD: 2 SERVINGS
PREPARATION TIME: 15 MINUTES, PLUS SOAKING TIME
COOKING TIME: NONE

INGREDIENTS:
1 medium ruby red grapefruit
1 medium orange
½ teaspoon brown sugar
4 medium pitted prunes
2 tablespoons plain nonfat yogurt

1. Halve the grapefruit and the orange. Using a serrated knife, remove the segments, working over a bowl to collect juices.
2. Put grapefruit and orange segments into a small bowl; sprinkle with brown sugar.
3. Add the prunes
4. Heat the reserved fruit juice and pour over the fruit. Cover and refrigerate at least 2 hours or overnight.
5. Serve topped with yogurt.

Estimated nutrients per serving:
Calories: 220
Total protein (grams): 3
Soy protein (grams): 0
Total carbohydrate (grams): 55
Total fat (grams): 0.5
Total fiber (grams): 5
Total fruit and vegetable (servings): 2

For prostate protection: *You can use this recipe as is.*

BREAKFAST ARAM

Flatbreads are used in many cultures. They are often spread with filling and rolled jelly-roll fashion to make sandwiches. Crackerbread, a type of flatbread, must be soaked to soften it before sandwich preparation. Soft flatbread is easier to use because it does not require soaking. If you're not going to serve the sandwiches right away, wrap them tightly in plastic wrap to keep them moist. Breakfast Aram is delicious when dunked in the fruit juices of the Citrus Delight, page 85.

YIELD: 2 SERVINGS
PREPARATION TIME: 10 MINUTES
COOKING TIME: NONE

INGREDIENTS:
   4 ounces nonfat cream cheese
   1 teaspoon honey
   1 tablespoon sliced almonds, toasted
   2 pieces soft flatbread, 12 inches square

1. In a small bowl, stir the cream cheese and honey until soft and spreadable. Add almonds and stir to combine.
2. Spread the mixture evenly on the flatbreads. Roll up.

Estimated nutrients per serving:
   Calories: 260
   Total protein (grams): 15
   Soy protein (grams): 0
   Total carbohydrate (grams): 40
   Total fat (grams): 4
   Total fiber (grams): 2
   Total fruit and vegetable (servings): none

For prostate protection: *For minimal dietary fat, use ½ instead of 1 tablespoon almonds.*

SOUPS AND STEWS

BASIC RECIPES

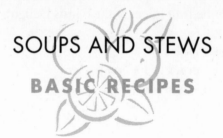

VEGETABLE STOCK

This nonfat stock can be used as an alternative to dehydrated or canned vegetable stock. It can be made in a large quantity and frozen in smaller amounts for use in many of the recipes in this book. The rich brown of the stock depends on sautéing the vegetables until they are deep golden brown in color. It smells great while you're cooking it.

YIELD: APPROXIMATELY 1 QUART
PREPARATION TIME: 10 MINUTES
COOKING TIME: 2 HOURS AND 10 MINUTES

INGREDIENTS:
   1 teaspoon olive oil
   ½ large onion, chopped
   2 large celery stalks, chopped
   1 large carrot, chopped
   ½ medium rutabaga, chopped
   5 cups water

1. In a saucepan, heat the olive oil over medium heat. Add onion and celery; cook for 5 minutes or until golden.
2. Add carrot and rutabaga. Continue to cook 5 minutes or longer, until all vegetables are deep golden brown in color.
3. Add water; bring to a boil. Reduce heat to low; cover and simmer for 2 hours.
4. Strain; discard vegetables. Refrigerate until cold. Remove any fat that has risen to the top.
5. Store in the refrigerator for as long as 5 days. Freeze for longer storage.

Estimated nutrients per cup:
Calories: 10
Total protein (grams): 0
Soy protein (grams): 0
Total carbohydrate (grams): 2
Total fat (grams): 0
Total fiber (grams): 0

For prostate protection: *You can use this recipe as is.*

VEGETABLE GRAVY

YIELD: 2½ CUPS
PREPARATION TIME: 5 MINUTES
COOKING TIME: 20 MINUTES

INGREDIENTS:
3 tablespoons cornstarch
2½ cups vegetable stock, homemade (page 88) or canned
¼ teaspoon salt

1. In a small bowl or teacup, combine the cornstarch and ¼ cup of the stock. Stir until no lumps remain.
2. Transfer to a medium saucepan, stir in the remainder of the stock, and bring to a boil over medium-high heat, stirring constantly.
3. Reduce to a low heat. Cook for 5 minutes, gently stirring the whole time.
4. Stir in salt.
5. Use in recipes as directed.

Estimated nutrients per 2 tablespoons:
Calories: 10
Total protein (grams): 0
Soy protein (grams): 0
Total carbohydrate (grams): 2
Total fat (grams): 0
Total fiber (grams): 0

For prostate protection: *You can use this recipe as is.*

BASIC WHITE SAUCE

This basic white sauce can be used in many recipes, such as broccoli soup or Eggs Florentine, page 65. Always stir thickened sauces gently — vigorous stirring will cause the sauce to lose its thickness.

YIELD: 1 CUP
PREPARATION TIME: 5 MINUTES
COOKING TIME: 10 MINUTES

INGREDIENTS:
  4 teaspoons cornstarch
  1 cup nonfat milk
  ⅛ teaspoon salt
  Pinch pepper
  Pinch nutmeg

1. In a small bowl or teacup, combine the cornstarch and 2 tablespoons of the milk. Stir until no lumps remain.
2. Transfer to a small saucepan, stir in the remainder of the milk, and bring to a boil over medium-high heat, stirring constantly.
3. Reduce to a low heat. Cook for 4 minutes, gently stirring the whole time.
4. Stir in salt, pepper, and nutmeg.
5. Use in recipes as directed.

Estimated nutrients per ¼ cup:
  Calories: 30
  Total protein (grams): 2
  Soy protein (grams): 0
  Total carbohydrate (grams): 5
  Total fat (grams): 0
  Total fiber (grams): 0

For prostate protection: You can use this recipe as is.

ASIAN

TOFU-MUSHROOM SOUP

This is a luncheon treat for mushroom fanciers. Although we have used three different types of mushrooms, the unique flavor of each one is retained.

YIELD: 2 SERVINGS, 2 CUPS EACH
PREPARATION TIME: 20 MINUTES, PLUS 20 MINUTES TO SOAK MUSHROOMS
COOKING TIME: 10 MINUTES

INGREDIENTS:

2 medium dried black mushrooms
¾ cup hot water
1½ cups vegetable stock, homemade (page 88) or canned
8 thin leek slices
¼ medium carrot, thinly sliced on the diagonal
1 cup chopped baby bok choy
2 medium button mushrooms, thinly sliced
1 large shiitake mushroom, thinly sliced
1 tablespoon miso
¼ teaspoon oyster sauce
¼ cup warm water
3 ounces extra-firm tofu, cut into small, thin pieces

1. Rinse dried mushrooms under cold water. Soak in the hot water for 20 minutes or until soft. Drain; slice mushrooms. Add soaking liquid to the vegetable stock in a saucepan; bring to a boil.
2. Wash the leek slices well to remove the dirt.
3. Add leeks, carrot, and bok choy to the saucepan. Cook for 5 minutes.
4. Add all mushrooms; return to a boil.
5. Dissolve miso and oyster sauce in ¼ cup warm water in a small bowl; add to saucepan.
6. Add tofu, return to a boil, and serve.

Estimated nutrients per serving:
Calories: 60
Total protein (grams): 6
Soy protein (grams): 4
Total carbohydrate (grams): 8
Total fat (grams): 1
Total fiber (grams): 3
Total fruit and vegetable (servings): 2½, including 1 serving
of cruciferous vegetable

For prostate protection: *You can use this recipe as is.*

BLACK MUSHROOM SOUP

The strong flavors of the two cruciferous vegetables, broccoli and turnip, and the black mushrooms combine to create an unusual and very tasty soup.

YIELD: 2 SERVINGS

PREPARATION TIME: 15 MINUTES, PLUS 20
MINUTES TO SOAK MUSHROOMS

COOKING TIME: 15 MINUTES

INGREDIENTS:
5 medium dried black mushrooms
1½ cups hot water
1 cup vegetable stock, homemade (page 88) or canned
2 medium green onions, sliced (include part of the green)
½ medium turnip, cut in matchstick-size pieces
½ cup broccoli florets, cut into small pieces
2 tablespoons miso
2 teaspoons sherry vinegar
1 teaspoon tamari soy sauce
¼ teaspoon chili oil
½ cup warm water
1 tablespoon thinly sliced green onion tops

1. Rinse dried mushrooms under cold water. Soak in the 1½ cups hot water for 20 minutes or until soft. Drain; slice mushrooms. Add soaking liquid to the vegetable stock in a saucepan; bring to a boil.
2. Add mushrooms, green onions, turnip, and broccoli to stock. Bring to a boil.
3. In a small bowl, combine miso, sherry vinegar, tamari sauce, and chili oil with the ½ cup warm water; add to soup.
4. Heat and serve, topped with sliced green onion tops.

Estimated nutrients per serving:
Calories: 70
Total protein (grams): 4
Soy protein (grams): 2
Total carbohydrate (grams): 11
Total fat (grams): 2
Total fiber (grams): 3
Total fruit and vegetable (servings): 2, including 1 serving of cruciferous vegetable

For prostate protection: *You can use this recipe as is.*

THAI SOUP

The coconut milk used in this recipe is made from nonfat milk and has to be prepared at least one day in advance. See recipe on page 221 for instructions. Preparing this soup is easy but takes last-minute juggling. It helps to read through all the instructions before starting to cook it.

YIELD: 2 SERVINGS
PREPARATION TIME: 15 MINUTES
COOKING TIME: 30 MINUTES

INGREDIENTS:
1½ cups vegetable stock, homemade (page 88) or canned
1 cup water
½ teaspoon freshly grated ginger
1 (2-inch) piece lemongrass, smashed
2 cloves roasted garlic, minced

1 or 2 small dried red chili peppers
1 medium carrot, thinly sliced on the diagonal
1½ cups chopped bok choy, stems and leaves
8 medium snow peas, ends and strings removed,
    thinly sliced on the diagonal
1 medium green onion, cut into 1-inch sections, then cut lengthwise
    into thin strips
¾ cup fresh green soybeans
2 ounces cooked baby shrimp
2 ounces Asian-style vermicelli noodles
½ cup coconut milk (page 221)
1 cup mung bean sprouts, blanched
2 tablespoons coarsely chopped cilantro leaves
2 wedges lime

1. In a large saucepan, combine stock, water, ginger, lemongrass, garlic, and dried chili peppers. Bring to a boil, reduce heat to very low, cover, and simmer gently for 20 minutes. Strain to remove the solid bits. Return broth to pan.
2. Meanwhile, in another large saucepan, bring 6 cups of water to a boil for the noodles.
3. Bring broth to a boil; add carrot and return to a boil. Add bok choy, snow peas, green onion, soybeans, and shrimp. Return to a boil, reduce heat, and keep warm.
4. Cook the noodles according to package directions. Drain noodles and add them to the soup. Add coconut milk. Stir well to combine.
5. Ladle into large individual soup or pasta bowls and top with mung bean sprouts and cilantro. Serve with lime wedges.

Estimated nutrients per serving:
Calories: 250
Total protein (grams): 20
Soy protein (grams): 8
Total carbohydrate (grams): 34
Total fat (grams): 5
Total fiber (grams): 5
Total fruit and vegetable (servings): 3, including 1 serving of cruciferous vegetable

For prostate protection: *To eliminate animal products, omit shrimp; make coconut milk with water instead of nonfat milk.*

LAOTIAN FISH SOUP

The wonderful taste of the broth in this soup develops from the infusion of the halibut, vegetables, and lemongrass. It is a satisfying meal in a bowl.

YIELD: 2 SERVINGS
PREPARATION TIME: 20 MINUTES
COOKING TIME: 30 MINUTES

INGREDIENTS:
  2 cups vegetable stock, homemade (page 88) or canned
  1 (1½-inch) piece lemongrass, smashed using the side of a knife
  1½ teaspoons fresh lemon juice
  6 cloves roasted garlic, minced
  ½ teaspoon fish sauce
  ¼ teaspoon hoisin sauce
  ⅛ teaspoon sesame oil
  ½ teaspoon sugar
  6 ounces halibut, cubed
  ½ medium carrot, thinly sliced on the diagonal
  1 cup broccoli florets
  2 small green onions, chopped
  ½ medium tomato, chopped
  ¾ cup fresh green soybeans
  2 tablespoons chopped cilantro
  2 cups cooked brown rice (page 178)

1. In a large saucepan, combine vegetable stock, lemongrass, lemon juice, garlic, fish sauce, hoisin sauce, sesame oil, and sugar. Bring to a boil, reduce heat, cover, and simmer gently for 20 minutes. Strain to remove the solid bits.
2. Return broth to pan and bring to a boil. Add fish, carrot, and broccoli. Reduce heat to medium and simmer for 8 minutes.
3. Add green onions, tomato, and soybeans. Heat for 2 minutes longer.
4. Top with cilantro; serve with brown rice.

Estimated nutrients per serving:
Calories: 420
Total protein (grams): 31

Soy protein (grams): 8
Total carbohydrate (grams): 59
Total fat (grams): 8
Total fiber (grams): 9
Total fruit and vegetable (servings): 2, including 1 serving of cruciferous vegetable

For prostate protection:

▪ *To increase lycopene, the prostate-healthy antioxidant and carotenoid that gives tomatoes their red color, use 1 instead of ½ medium tomato.*

▪ *To eliminate animal products, omit halibut.*

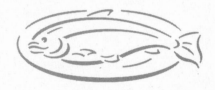

NEW AMERICAN

KALE AND CUCUMBER SOUP

This light, refreshing soup can also be chilled and served cold. When you're making it, consider doubling the recipe so you have some to refrigerate and take to work in a thermos. One taste judge wrote, "I drank it chilled. I especially love the subtle taste of cucumber and garlic, which leaves you feeling invigorated. How great that such a delicious soup actually contains kale, which is a nutritious cruciferous vegetable."

YIELD: 2 SERVINGS
PREPARATION TIME: 15 MINUTES
COOKING TIME: 20 MINUTES

INGREDIENTS:
    8 large leaves kale
    ¼ teaspoon olive oil
    1 medium cucumber, peeled
    1 clove roasted garlic, minced
    2 tablespoons toasted slivered almonds
    ¼ teaspoon salt
    ¼ cup water
    ½ cup plain nonfat yogurt
    1 tablespoon plain nonfat yogurt
    2 fresh dill sprigs

1. Wash kale thoroughly. Remove and discard stems; shred leaves.
2. Steam kale for 10 minutes, or until soft. Add oil to kale.
3. Meanwhile, puree cucumber, garlic, and almonds together in a food processor or blender.
4. Add cooked kale and salt; puree until blended.
5. Add water and the ½ cup yogurt; mix thoroughly.
6. To serve cold: Refrigerate for at least 2 hours or overnight. Divide between 2 bowls and top each with ½ tablespoon nonfat yogurt and a dill sprig.

7. To serve hot: Transfer soup to saucepan and heat, stirring, until hot but not boiling. Divide between 2 bowls and top each with ½ tablespoon nonfat yogurt and a dill sprig.

Estimated nutrients per serving:
 Calories: 140
 Total protein (grams): 8
 Soy protein (grams): 0
 Total carbohydrate (grams): 14
 Total fat (grams): 6
 Total fiber (grams): 3
 Total fruit and vegetable (servings): 3, including 2 servings of cruciferous vegetable

For prostate protection:
 ■ *To eliminate animal products, replace the ½ cup yogurt with ½ cup nonfat soy milk and omit yogurt topping.*
 ■ *For minimal dietary fat, omit almonds.*

BLACK BEAN AND MUSHROOM STEW WITH PARMESAN POLENTA

This recipe got rave reviews when Rita served it at a festive holiday meal. You can make this stew ahead of time and assemble it in a casserole dish to be reheated at serving time. To do this, spread the cooked polenta evenly in a nonstick 1½-quart baking dish. Spoon mushroom stew over polenta, cover, and refrigerate. Bake, covered, in a 350-degree oven for 30 minutes or until hot. Regular cornmeal can be used in place of the polenta, which is coarsely ground cornmeal.

YIELD: 4 SERVINGS
PREPARATION TIME: 30 MINUTES
COOKING TIME: 30 MINUTES

INGREDIENTS:
 For polenta:
 3 cups boiling water
 ¼ teaspoon salt

1 cup polenta (coarsely ground cornmeal)
1 tablespoon freshly grated Parmesan cheese

For stew:
4 large shiitake mushrooms
4 large button mushrooms
½ medium onion, chopped
2 cloves roasted garlic, minced
1 (15-ounce) can black beans, drained, not rinsed
2 teaspoons tomato paste
½ cup vegetable stock, homemade (page 88) or canned
½ teaspoon salt

1. In a large, heavy saucepan, bring water and salt to a boil. Gradually add polenta in a steady stream, stirring continuously with a wooden spoon. Reduce to a very low heat. Cook 30 minutes longer, stirring frequently. If polenta becomes too thick to stir, add hot water, a tablespoon at a time. Polenta should be very thick but still stirable. Stir in Parmesan cheese.
2. Meanwhile, remove stems from shiitake mushrooms; slice shiitake and button mushrooms.
3. Place mushrooms, onion, and garlic in a large nonstick frying pan over medium heat and cook for 15 minutes.
4. Add beans, tomato paste, stock, and salt to mushrooms; heat until boiling.
5. Spoon polenta onto serving plates; ladle stew over the polenta.

Estimated nutrients per serving:
Calories: 230
Total protein (grams): 9
Soy protein (grams): 0
Total carbohydrate (grams): 46
Total fat (grams): 1.5
Total fiber (grams): 7
Total fruit and vegetable (servings): 1

For prostate protection: *To eliminate animal products, replace Parmesan cheese with chopped Italian parsley.*

THREE-BEAN CHILI

Christmas lima beans retain their unique colorful speckles even when cooked. They are not available canned. Cook them like you would any other dried bean (see basic bean recipe, page 181).

YIELD: 5 SERVINGS, 1½ CUPS EACH
PREPARATION TIME: 20 MINUTES
COOKING TIME: 15 MINUTES

INGREDIENTS:

1 teaspoon olive oil
1 medium onion, chopped
2 cups cooked Christmas lima beans
1 (15-ounce) can black beans, drained, not rinsed
1 (15-ounce) can soybeans, drained, not rinsed;
   or 2 cups cooked mature soybeans (page 181)
1 medium turnip, cubed
2 stalks celery, coarsely chopped
3 cups vegetable stock, homemade (page 88) or canned
1 (3½-ounce) can diced green chilies
½ cup tomato sauce
1 teaspoon red chili powder
1 teaspoon cumin powder

1. In a large pot, heat olive oil over medium-high heat. Add onion; cook for 15 minutes, until onion is deep golden.
2. Add all other ingredients; stir gently.
3. Bring to a boil. Reduce heat and simmer for 10 to 15 minutes, until vegetables are soft.

Estimated nutrients per serving:

Calories: 500
Total protein (grams): 37
Soy protein (grams): 9
Total carbohydrate (grams): 60
Total fat (grams): 11
Total fiber (grams): 22
Total fruit and vegetable (servings): 1, including ½ serving of cruciferous vegetable

For prostate protection: *To increase lycopene — the prostate-healthy anti-oxidant and carotenoid that gives tomatoes their red color — use 2 cups vegetable stock and 1½ cups tomato sauce instead of the stock and tomato sauce in the recipe.*

BLACK BEAN AND RICE SOUP

Beans and rice have been enjoyed in combination by people of many cultures for centuries. We developed this recipe to incorporate soy protein, in the form of tempeh, and rutabaga, a cruciferous vegetable, into a soup that is delicious and easy to prepare.

YIELD: 4 SERVINGS
PREPARATION TIME: 20 MINUTES
COOKING TIME: 30 MINUTES

INGREDIENTS:
1 teaspoon olive oil
¼ medium onion, chopped
2 cloves roasted garlic, minced
1 (15-ounce) can black beans, drained, not rinsed
½ cup cooked brown rice (page 178)
4 ounces soy tempeh, crumbled
2 cups finely shredded collard greens
1 medium rutabaga, finely diced
1½ cups vegetable stock, homemade (page 88) or canned
¼ teaspoon salt
⅛ teaspoon pepper
⅛ teaspoon cumin powder
⅛ teaspoon oregano

1. In a large pot, heat olive oil over medium-high heat. Add onion and garlic and cook for 15 minutes, until onion is deep golden.
2. Add all other ingredients except spices. Bring to a boil and simmer for 10 minutes.
3. Add spices and simmer for an additional 5 minutes.

Estimated nutrients per serving:
Calories: 260
Total protein (grams): 15
Soy protein (grams): 5
Total carbohydrate (grams): 44
Total fat (grams): 3
Total fiber (grams): 11
Total fruit and vegetable (servings): 1½, including 1½ servings of cruciferous vegetable

For prostate protection: *For minimal dietary fat, use ½ instead of 1 teaspoon olive oil.*

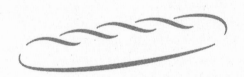

MEDITERRANEAN

MINESTRONE

Don't be discouraged by the number of ingredients in this hearty soup. It goes together quickly and makes a large quantity to enjoy for several meals. As with most soups, this is best made ahead of time to let the flavors develop.

YIELD: 6 SERVINGS
PREPARATION TIME: 30 MINUTES
COOKING TIME: 1 HOUR TOTAL

INGREDIENTS:
2 tablespoons olive oil
½ medium onion, chopped
2 stalks celery with leaves, chopped
2 cloves roasted garlic, minced
1 medium potato, scrubbed and diced
1 medium rutabaga, peeled and diced
1 large carrot, peeled and diced
4 cups vegetable stock, homemade (page 88) or canned
4 cups water
2 tablespoons tomato paste
1 cup French beans, trimmed and cut in half
1 cup chopped collard greens
1 cup shredded cabbage
1 cup uncooked large pasta shells
1 (15-ounce) can garbanzo beans, drained, not rinsed
1 (15-ounce) can red kidney beans, drained, not rinsed
2 cups fresh green soybeans
½ teaspoon salt
¼ teaspoon pepper
½ teaspoon oregano

1. Heat olive oil in a large, heavy saucepan.
2. Add onion, celery, and garlic; sauté for about 5 minutes, until vegetables are lightly browned.

3. Add potato, rutabaga, and carrot; continue cooking for an additional 5 minutes.
4. Add stock, water, and tomato paste; bring to a boil.
5. Add French beans, collard greens, and cabbage.
6. When soup returns to a boil, add pasta. Simmer for 20 minutes.
7. Add garbanzo and kidney beans and soybeans and seasonings. Cook for 2 minutes longer.

Estimated nutrients per serving:
Calories: 440
Total protein (grams): 24
Soy protein (grams): 7
Total carbohydrate (grams): 68
Total fat (grams): 11
Total fiber (grams): 16
Total fruit and vegetable (servings): 2, including 1 serving of cruciferous vegetable

For prostate protection:
■ *To increase lycopene (the prostate-healthy antioxidant and carotenoid that gives tomatoes their red color), use 4 cups tomato juice instead of the water.*
■ *For minimal dietary fat, use 1 instead of 2 tablespoons olive oil.*

WHITE BEAN STEW

This is a deliciously rich and satisfying stew that will be ever popular with family and friends on a chilly day. This was developed from a recipe Barbara's father made to serve on Sunday evenings by the fire.

YIELD: 6 SERVINGS
PREPARATION TIME: 30 MINUTES
COOKING TIME: 30 MINUTES

INGREDIENTS:
2 tablespoons olive oil
½ medium onion, chopped
4 cloves roasted garlic, minced
2 cups vegetable stock, homemade (page 88) or canned

1 medium rutabaga, peeled and diced
½ cup cubed butternut squash
2 cups broccoli florets
1 (15-ounce) can small white beans, including liquid
1 (15-ounce) can soybeans, drained, not rinsed;
   or 2 cups cooked mature soybeans (page 181)
1 tablespoon chopped Italian parsley
½ teaspoon cumin powder
⅛ teaspoon pepper

1. Heat oil in a large saucepan over medium heat. Add onion and garlic; sauté for about 10 minutes, until onion is golden.
2. Add stock, rutabaga, and squash. Bring to a boil, cover, reduce heat, and cook for about 15 minutes, until vegetables are soft.
3. Add broccoli; return to a boil.
4. Add beans and seasonings. Heat and serve.

Estimated nutrients per serving:
Calories: 310
Total protein (grams): 21
Soy protein (grams): 12
Total carbohydrate (grams): 35
Total fat (grams): 11
Total fiber (grams): 11
Total fruit and vegetable (servings): 1, including 1 serving of cruciferous vegetable

For prostate protection: *For minimal dietary fat, use 1 instead of 2 tablespoons olive oil.*

POTATO-KALE SOUP

This is a scrumptious soup with a unique flavor that has become a comfort food for us.

YIELD: 2 SERVINGS
PREPARATION TIME: 10 MINUTES
COOKING TIME: 40 MINUTES

INGREDIENTS:

2 medium russet potatoes, peeled and quartered
2 cups packed cooked kale (page 192)
¼ teaspoon salt
⅛ teaspoon pepper
2 teaspoons olive oil
¼ cup vegetable stock, homemade (page 88) or canned

1. Boil potatoes until soft; drain.
2. Put potatoes in food processor or blender; puree.
3. Add cooked kale, salt, pepper, olive oil, and vegetable stock to blender. Blend until smooth.
4. Add additional stock if a thinner consistency is desired.
5. Return to saucepan and heat.

Estimated nutrients per serving:
Calories: 190
Total protein (grams): 6
Soy protein (grams): 0
Total carbohydrate (grams): 32
Total fat (grams): 5
Total fiber (grams): 5
Total fruit and vegetable (servings): 2, including 1 serving of cruciferous vegetable

For prostate protection: *For minimal dietary fat, use 1 instead of 2 teaspoons olive oil.*

VEGETABLE AND BEAN RAGOUT OVER COUSCOUS

Couscous is a staple in many Moroccan meals. This nontraditional ragout uses garbanzo beans and soybeans as a protein source. The nutty flavor of these beans gives richness to the vegetable-based recipe.

YIELD: 4
PREPARATION TIME: 15 MINUTES
COOKING TIME: 15 MINUTES

INGREDIENTS
1½ cups water
1½ cups couscous

4 teaspoons olive oil

½ medium onion, chopped

4 cups finely shredded kale

1 large turnip, peeled and chopped

½ large sweet red pepper, stems, seeds, and membranes removed; sliced

1 cup canned garbanzo beans

1 (15-ounce) can soybeans, drained; or 2 cups cooked mature
   soybeans (page 181)

½ teaspoon coriander

½ teaspoon cardamom

¼ teaspoon cinnamon

½ teaspoon turmeric

¼ teaspoon salt

2 cups hot water

1. Bring the 1½ cups water to a boil in a small saucepan. Remove
   from heat. Stir in couscous. Set aside; keep warm.
2. In a medium saucepan, heat olive oil over medium heat; add
   onion, kale, turnip, and red pepper. Cook for 5 minutes, until soft.
3. Stir in garbanzo beans and soybeans, coriander, cardamom, cinnamon, tumeric, salt, and the hot water.
4. Bring to a boil. Reduce heat and simmer for 5 minutes to heat
   through.
5. Fluff couscous with a fork. Serve ragout over couscous.

Estimated nutrients per serving:

Calories: 550

Total protein (grams): 31

Soy protein (grams): 18

Total carbohydrate (grams): 75

Total fat (grams): 17

Total fiber (grams): 17

Total fruit and vegetable (servings): 2, including 1 serving of cruciferous vegetable

For prostate protection:

▪ To increase lycopene, add 1 medium tomato, chopped, in step 2.
▪ For minimal dietary fat, use 2 instead of 4 teaspoons olive oil.

BOUILLABAISSE

Bouillabaisse is the most famous of the fish stews of the Mediterranean region. In this recipe we have used halibut, sole, mussels, clams, and shrimp. Vary the fish selection as you desire each time you make it. A big steaming bowlful of this hearty stew is great for lunch or dinner any day, any season.

YIELD: 2 SERVINGS
PREPARATION TIME: 30 MINUTES
COOKING TIME: 20 MINUTES

INGREDIENTS:
½ cup thinly sliced leeks
2 tablespoons olive oil
½ cup chopped celery
¼ cup sweet red pepper slices
½ cup small diced rutabaga
4 cloves roasted garlic, minced
1 cup chopped canned tomatoes with juice
2 cups vegetable stock, homemade (page 88) or canned
½ cup small broccoli florets
4 ounces halibut
4 ounces petrale sole or flounder
4 mussels
4 clams
4 medium shrimp
2 bay leaves, crushed
¼ teaspoon salt
⅛ teaspoon pepper
¼ teaspoon dried basil
¼ teaspoon saffron threads
1 teaspoon grated orange peel

1. Wash the leeks thoroughly to remove grit.
2. In a medium saucepan, heat olive oil over medium-high heat; add leeks, celery, red pepper, rutabaga, and garlic. Cook for 3 minutes, until leeks are golden brown.
3. Add tomatoes and vegetable stock; bring to a boil.
4. Add broccoli, halibut, and sole. Cook for 5 minutes.

5. Wash mussels and clams thoroughly; scrub shells with a brush.
6. Add mussels and clams to the stew. Cook for 3 to 5 minutes, until the shells open.
7. Add shrimp and seasonings. Cook for 1 minute longer. Remove from heat. Do not overcook.

Estimated nutrients per serving:
Calories: 370
Total protein (grams): 36
Soy protein (grams): 0
Total carbohydrate (grams): 20
Total fat (grams): 16
Total fiber (grams): 5
Total fruit and vegetable (servings): 3, including 1 serving of cruciferous vegetable

For prostate protection: *For minimal dietary fat, use 1 instead of 2 tablespoons olive oil.*

RATATOUILLE

This is a classic vegetable stew in which the vegetables are cooked until they are very soft. Although it requires a bit of time, it is easy to prepare and the result is worthwhile. It is very versatile and is delicious hot, cold, or at room temperature.

YIELD: 4 SERVINGS
PREPARATION TIME: ½ HOUR, PLUS SALTING TIME
COOKING TIME: 45 MINUTES

INGREDIENTS:
1 large eggplant
1 tablespoon salt
3 tablespoons extra-virgin olive oil
½ large onion, chopped
2 cloves roasted garlic, minced
1 large rutabaga, peeled and thinly sliced
½ large green pepper, sliced
1 medium zucchini, sliced

¼ teaspoon pepper
½ teaspoon dried basil
½ teaspoon dried oregano
1½ cups fresh green soybeans
1½ cups canned diced tomatoes
2 tablespoons water

1. Peel the eggplant and cut into ½-inch slices. Spread on a cookie sheet lined with a paper towel. Sprinkle with half of the salt. When tiny droplets of water form on the surface of the eggplant, turn the eggplant slices over and sprinkle with remaining salt. Let stand 1 hour.
2. Rinse each slice well with cold water; drain.
3. Heat oil over medium heat in a large nonstick skillet that has a lid. Add onion and garlic; cook 5 minutes.
4. Add rutabaga, green pepper, and zucchini slices. Cook another 5 minutes, stirring gently; sprinkle pepper, basil, and oregano evenly over the mixture.
5. Add eggplant in a layer over the top. Do not stir. Cover with the lid, reduce heat to low, and cook for 30 minutes, until eggplant is very soft.
6. Add the soybeans, tomatoes, and water; stir just to mix. Cook uncovered over low heat for 15 minutes longer.

Estimated nutrients per serving:
Calories: 330
Total protein (grams): 13
Soy protein (grams): 7
Total carbohydrate (grams): 36
Total fat (grams): 15
Total fiber (grams): 13
Total fruit and vegetable (servings): 3, including ½ serving of cruciferous vegetable

For prostate protection: *For minimal dietary fat, use 2 instead of 3 tablespoons olive oil.*

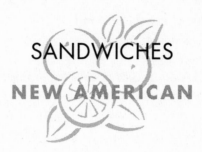

SANDWICHES
NEW AMERICAN

OPEN-FACE LENTIL-NUT LOAF SANDWICH

Some people cook a turkey at Thanksgiving just to have leftovers for sandwiches. We cook this lentil loaf and serve it hot as an entrée (smothered with our delicious vegetable gravy, page 89) just to have leftovers for this sandwich. The loaf in this recipe yields 8 portions.

YIELD: LOAF: 8 PORTIONS; SANDWICH: 1 SERVING
PREPARATION TIME: 30 MINUTES FOR THE LENTIL
   LOAF; 10 MINUTES TO PREPARE THE SANDWICH
COOKING TIME: 45 MINUTES FOR THE LENTIL LOAF,
   NONE FOR THE SANDWICH

INGREDIENTS:
For lentil loaf:
¾ cup boiling water
1 cup bulgur (cracked wheat)
2 cups cooked lentils (page 179)
2 slices French bread, broken into pieces
4 ounces soy tempeh, crumbled
½ medium onion, roasted and chopped
¼ cup chopped pecans, toasted
2 medium dried figs, sliced
¼ cup tomato sauce
½ cup vegetable stock, homemade (page 88) or canned
½ teaspoon salt
⅛ teaspoon pepper

For sandwich:

1 (6-inch-long) portion baguette or roll
2 tablespoons plain nonfat yogurt
1 (1-inch) slice lentil loaf
1 slice sun-dried tomato packed in olive oil, drained and chopped
1 tablespoon chopped green onion

To prepare lentil loaf:

Preheat oven to 350 degrees.

1. Pour boiling water over bulgur in a small bowl; set aside for at least 15 minutes.
2. In a large bowl, mix all other lentil loaf ingredients. Mix in bulgur.
3. Spoon mixture into a 4×8-inch loaf pan that has been lined with foil.
4. Bake at 350 degrees for 45 minutes.
5. Remove loaf from pan; gently remove foil. Let stand 15 minutes before cutting.

To prepare sandwich:

1. Cut baguette or roll in half lengthwise; spread with yogurt.
2. Cut lentil loaf slice to cover the surface of the baguette or roll.
3. Sprinkle with tomato and green onion.

Estimated nutrients per serving:

Calories: 330
Total protein (grams): 14
Soy protein (grams): 3
Total carbohydrate (grams): 56
Total fat (grams): 8
Total fiber (grams): 11
Total fruit and vegetable (servings): 1

For prostate protection:

■ *For minimal dietary fat, omit pecans; use 2 slices fresh tomato instead of sun-dried tomato.*
■ *To eliminate animal products, use silken tofu instead of yogurt.*

SMOKED TOFU SANDWICH

This sandwich goes together quickly from ingredients you're likely to have on hand. Substitute whole wheat bread for the rolls if you like.

Smoked tofu has the texture and consistency of cheese. A cheese cutter works well to slice the tofu into thin slices. One of our taste judges said that this is a very delicious, crunchy, refreshing sandwich. He especially liked the smoked tofu with the red onion, lettuce, and tomato.

YIELD: 2 SANDWICHES
PREPARATION TIME: 10 MINUTES
COOKING TIME: NONE

INGREDIENTS
2 crusty whole wheat rolls
2 tablespoons plain nonfat yogurt
½ teaspoon extra-virgin olive oil
4 ounces extra-firm smoked tofu, thinly sliced
4 thick slices tomato
2 leaves romaine lettuce
2 thin slices red onion
¼ cup radish slices
1 cup broccoli florets, blanched

1. Slice rolls in half lengthwise.
2. Mix together the yogurt and olive oil. Spread both cut sides of rolls with mixture.
3. Add tofu, tomato slices, lettuce leaf, and onion to the bottom half of each roll.
4. Cover with top half.
5. Serve on a plate with radish slices and broccoli florets.

Estimated nutrients per serving:
Calories: 150
Total protein (grams): 8
Soy protein (grams): 3
Total carbohydrate (grams): 22
Total fat (grams): 4
Total fiber (grams): 4
Total fruit and vegetable (servings): 2, including 1 serving of cruciferous vegetable

For prostate protection:
■ *To eliminate animal products, use silken tofu instead of yogurt.*
■ *For minimal dietary fat, use ¼ instead of ½ teaspoon olive oil.*

TUNA MELT

Here is a low-fat version of the flavorful traditional tuna melt, which has been modified to incorporate tofu as the source of soy protein. In this recipe, the vegetables are cooked briefly to enhance their flavor. This step can be omitted for a quicker preparation. One taste judge said she definitely wouldn't eliminate this step because the lightly cooked peppers and green onion add a wonderful crunchy texture.

The thinly sliced and melted low-fat cheddar and yogurt are excellent substitutions for the traditional fatty cheese and mayonnaise.

YIELD: 2 SANDWICHES

PREPARATION TIME: 10 MINUTES

COOKING TIME: 3 MINUTES (BE CAREFUL NOT
  TO LEAVE IT TOO LONG IN THE BROILER,
  AS THE CHEESE WILL BURN)

INGREDIENTS:
  ½ teaspoon olive oil
  2 tablespoons finely chopped green bell pepper
  2 tablespoons finely chopped sweet red pepper
  1 tablespoon finely chopped green onion
  1 (6-ounce) can water-packed albacore tuna, drained
  2 tablespoons plain nonfat yogurt
  ½ teaspoon olive oil
  3½ ounces savory baked tofu, thinly sliced
  4 slices French bread
  2 ounces low-fat cheddar cheese, thinly sliced

Preheat broiler.
  1. Heat olive oil over medium heat in a small skillet. Add peppers and onion; cook for 5 minutes.
  2. Combine tuna, yogurt, and olive oil in a small bowl. Add vegetables and mix.
  3. Layer the tofu evenly on two slices of bread, spread the tuna mix on the tofu, and cover evenly with the cheese.
  4. Place the open sandwiches on a cookie sheet and put briefly under preheated broiler to melt the cheese.

5. Top the sandwiches with the other slices of bread and return to broiler to toast the bread.

6. Turn sandwiches over; return to broiler briefly to toast the other side.

Estimated nutrients per serving:
Calories: 390
Total protein (grams): 38
Soy protein (grams): 3
Total carbohydrate (grams): 39
Total fat (grams): 10
Total fiber (grams): 3
Total fruit and vegetable (servings): none

For prostate protection: *This recipe cannot be modified to meet the prostate cancer recommendations.*

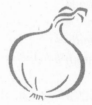

MEDITERRANEAN

PITA BREAD SANDWICH

Feel free to add lots more red pepper, cabbage, or parsley; or try it with other fresh vegetables. In this sandwich, shredded cabbage replaces the predictable lettuce. It adds crunch and a refreshing flavor. And as an added bonus, it's a cruciferous vegetable.

YIELD: 2 SERVINGS

PREPARATION TIME: 10 MINUTES

COOKING TIME: NONE

INGREDIENTS:

2 pita breads
½ cup soybean hummus (page 182)
¼ cup chopped sweet red pepper
1 cup shredded green cabbage
¼ cup plain nonfat yogurt
2 tablespoons sliced black olives
2 tablespoons chopped Italian parsley

1. Cut pita breads in half, or cut a small section from one edge to make a pocket.
2. Spread hummus on the inside bottom part of the pita. Fill the pita pocket with red pepper and cabbage.
3. Spread yogurt over peppers and cabbage. Sprinkle evenly with olives and parsley.

Estimated nutrients per serving:

Calories: 230
Total protein (grams): 12
Soy protein (grams): 7
Total carbohydrate (grams): 26
Total fat (grams): 10
Total fiber (grams): 6
Total fruit and vegetable (servings): 1, including 1 serving of cruciferous vegetable

For prostate protection:
- *To increase lycopene, add ½ cup chopped tomato in step 2.*
- *For minimal dietary fat, use 1 instead of 2 tablespoons sliced olives.*

GREEK SANDWICH

This is so good! When Barbara made it the first time, we were delighted at how good it was. We have made it several more times for picnics with friends in the hills of Oakland overlooking the beautiful San Francisco Bay.

YIELD: 2 SERVINGS

PREPARATION TIME: 10 MINUTES

COOKING TIME: 3 MINUTES

INGREDIENTS:
  2 (5-inch-diameter) crusty rolls
  ¼ cup silken tofu
  1 tablespoon packed soy protein powder
  2 teaspoons lemon juice
  1 teaspoon extra-virgin olive oil
  ⅛ teaspoon tarragon
  1½ tablespoons chopped walnuts
  ¼ medium red Anjou pear, chopped
  ½ tablespoon finely chopped green onion
  ¼ cup shredded romaine lettuce
  ½ cup crumbled reduced-fat feta cheese

Preheat oven to 350 degrees.
1. Cut rolls in half lengthwise but do not separate. Place in oven 3 minutes.
2. In a small bowl, combine tofu, soy protein powder, lemon juice, olive oil, and tarragon. Mix well. Stir in walnuts, pear, and green onion.
3. Separate rolls in half. Remove some of the dough from the center of each half to make a well.
4. Put tofu mixture into the bottom of each roll. Spread evenly to within ½ inch of the edge.
5. Top with lettuce and feta cheese. Cover with top of roll.

Estimated nutrients per serving:
Calories: 310
Total protein (grams): 16
Soy protein (grams): 6
Total carbohydrate (grams): 28
Total fat (grams): 17
Total fiber (grams): 3
Total fruit and vegetable (servings): ½

For prostate protection: *For minimal dietary fat, use ½ instead of 1 teaspoon olive oil, and 1 instead of 1½ tablespoons chopped walnuts.*

ARAM SANDWICH

On several occasions we have prepared these sandwiches ahead, wrapped them in plastic wrap, and put them in the refrigerator to see if they keep well for serving the next day. Our experiment has never been successful. The sandwiches vanish overnight! In the morning, Rita's son, Ryan, thanks her for leaving "those great rolled-up sandwiches" for a late-night snack.

YIELD: 2 SERVINGS

PREPARATION TIME: 20 MINUTES, PLUS 1 HOUR OF
   STANDING TIME FOR EGGPLANT

COOKING TIME: 5 MINUTES

INGREDIENTS:
   1 medium eggplant
   2 teaspoons salt
   4 ounces nonfat cream cheese
   2 tablespoons packed soy protein powder
   2 cloves roasted garlic, crushed
   ½ teaspoon olive oil
   1 tablespoon plain nonfat yogurt
   3 leaves fresh basil, chopped
   1½ tablespoons olive oil
   1 cup shredded cabbage
   ½ cup roasted red pepper, sliced

1 cup peeled cucumber, chopped
2 pieces soft flatbread, 12 inches square

1. Peel the eggplant and cut into ¼-inch slices. Spread on a cookie sheet lined with a paper towel. Sprinkle with half of the salt. When tiny droplets of water form on the surface of the eggplant, turn the eggplant slices over and sprinkle with remaining salt. Let stand 1 hour.
2. Meanwhile, stir the cream cheese until soft and spreadable. Stir in soy protein powder until smooth. Add garlic, the ½ teaspoon olive oil, yogurt, and basil; mix until smooth. Set aside.
3. Rinse the eggplant slices under cold water to remove salt. Drain. Chop eggplant coarsely.
4. In a skillet, heat the 1½ tablespoons olive oil over medium heat; add eggplant and cabbage. Cook 5 minutes or until soft, stirring occasionally. Transfer to a bowl to cool.
5. Stir in the red pepper and cucumber.
6. Spread the cream cheese mixture evenly on the flatbreads. Cover with vegetable mixture and roll tightly.
7. Cut into slices or serve as "logs."

Estimated nutrients per serving:
    Calories: 410
    Total protein (grams): 26
    Soy protein (grams): 8
    Total carbohydrate (grams): 62
    Total fat (grams): 9
    Total fiber (grams): 10
    Total fruit and vegetable (servings): 4, including 1 serving of cruciferous
        vegetable

For prostate protection: *For minimal dietary fat, use 1 instead of 1½ tablespoons olive oil in step 4.*

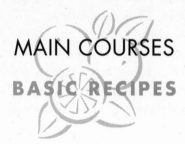

MAIN COURSES
BASIC RECIPES

FRESH PAPAYA AND MANGO CHUTNEY

Since this should be served cold, prepare it ahead of time to allow plenty of time for cooling. This keeps well in the refrigerator and is great to have on hand for use with curries.

YIELD: 2 CUPS
PREPARATION TIME: 10 MINUTES
COOKING TIME: 30 MINUTES

INGREDIENTS:
½ cup malt vinegar
½ cup water
¼ cup apple juice concentrate
2 cloves roasted garlic, minced
½ teaspoon freshly grated ginger
⅛ teaspoon red pepper flakes
1 cup chopped mango
1 cup chopped papaya
1 small Granny Smith apple, peeled and chopped
1 tablespoon raisins

1. In a medium saucepan, combine vinegar, water, apple juice concentrate, garlic, ginger, and red pepper flakes. Bring to a boil.
2. Add mango, papaya, and apple. Return to a boil, reduce heat, and simmer gently, uncovered, for 25 minutes.
3. Remove from heat; add raisins and let cool.

Estimated nutrients per ¼ cup:
　Calories: 45
　Total protein (grams): 0
　Soy protein (grams): 0
　Total carbohydrate (grams): 12
　Total fat (grams): 0
　Total fiber (grams): 1
　Total fruit and vegetable (servings): 1

For prostate protection: *You can use this recipe as is.*

MINT CHUTNEY

Prepare this ahead to allow plenty of time for the flavors to develop. As with all chutneys, Mint Chutney keeps well in the refrigerator.

YIELD: 1 CUP
PREPARATION TIME: 10 MINUTES
COOKING TIME: NONE

INGREDIENTS:
　1 cup packed mint leaves
　2 tablespoons malt vinegar
　½ tablespoon water
　2 tablespoons brown sugar
　1 medium Granny Smith apple, peeled and cored
　2 tablespoons chopped onion

1. Put all ingredients in a blender and process to form a pulp.
2. Serve with curries.

Estimated nutrients per ¼ cup:
　Calories: 40
　Total protein (grams): 0
　Soy protein (grams): 0
　Total carbohydrate (grams): 9

Total fat (grams): 0
Total fiber (grams): 1
Total fruit and vegetable (servings): none

For prostate protection: *You can use this recipe as is.*

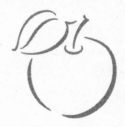

ASIAN

MIXED VEGETABLE STIR-FRY

Rita prepared this as one of the recipes for my appearance on the *Oprah Winfrey Show* for *The Breast Cancer Prevention Diet* book. It was a big hit.

YIELD: 2 SERVINGS
PREPARATION TIME: 15 MINUTES
COOKING TIME: 15 MINUTES

INGREDIENTS:
    ¼ teaspoon canola oil
    ½ cup broccoli florets (grape-size pieces)
    ½ cup cauliflower florets (grape-size pieces)
    10 medium snow peas
    ¼ medium sweet red pepper, sliced
    2 medium green onions, chopped
    ¼ cup sliced water chestnuts
    6 drops chili oil
    6 drops tamari soy sauce
    ¼ teaspoon freshly grated ginger
    2 ounces extra-firm tofu, cubed
    2 cups cooked brown rice (page 178)

1. Put canola oil in a large skillet or wok. Heat over medium heat.
2. Add broccoli and cauliflower and cook about 5 minutes, stirring constantly.
3. Add snow peas, red pepper, green onions, and water chestnuts. Cook about 5 minutes longer, stirring constantly.
4. Add chili oil, soy sauce, and ginger and mix thoroughly into vegetables.
5. Add tofu. Continue cooking for about 2 to 3 minutes, just to heat tofu. Stir gently.
6. Serve over brown rice.

Estimated nutrients per serving:
Calories: 270
Total protein (grams): 9
Soy protein (grams): 2
Total carbohydrate (grams): 54
Total fat (grams): 3
Total fiber (grams): 7
Total fruit and vegetable (servings): 2, including 1 serving of cruciferous vegetable

For prostate protection: *You can use this recipe as is.*

MU SHU VEGETABLES

Look for mu shu wrappers, called "pancakes," in Asian food markets or the produce section of a grocery store. If you can't find them, substitute small flour tortillas. The sweet and pungent plum sauce gives a characteristic flavor to this dish.

YIELD: 2 SERVINGS
PREPARATION TIME: 20 MINUTES
COOKING TIME: 20 MINUTES

INGREDIENTS:
1 medium dried black mushroom
½ cup hot water
2 teaspoons cornstarch
½ teaspoon freshly grated ginger
6 mu shu wrappers (pancakes)
½ teaspoon canola oil
½ cup chopped onion
½ cup chopped cabbage
½ cup chopped bok choy stems and leaves
½ cup shredded carrot
1 cup mung bean sprouts
5 ounces extra-firm tofu, drained and sliced
2 tablespoons plum sauce
1 medium green onion, thinly sliced

Preheat oven to 350 degrees.

1. Rinse mushroom under cold water. In a small bowl soak the mushroom in the hot water for 20 minutes or until soft.
2. Drain mushroom, saving liquid. Slice mushroom very thinly. Set aside.
3. Put the cornstarch in a small bowl; add 3 tablespoons of the reserved mushroom liquid. Stir to a thin paste; add remaining reserved liquid and ginger. Stir and set aside.
4. Wrap the mu shu wrappers in foil. Place in preheated oven while you prepare the vegetables.
5. In a large nonstick skillet, heat canola oil over medium heat; add onion. Cook for 10 minutes, until onion is soft. Add cabbage, bok choy, carrot, and reserved mushroom. Cook 5 minutes longer, stirring occasionally.
6. Add bean sprouts; stir to mix. Pour in cornstarch liquid; stir mixture constantly for 3 minutes or until sauce is thick. Add tofu and stir gently to mix. Cook for 2 minutes longer.
7. To serve, place the vegetables in a serving bowl and keep the pancakes warm. To assemble them, spread plum sauce and sprinkle green onion on a pancake. Place vegetable mixture along the center of the pancake; wrap to enclose the mixture.

Estimated nutrients per serving:

Calories: 330
Total protein (grams): 13
Soy protein (grams): 5
Total carbohydrate (grams): 60
Total fat (grams): 4.5
Total fiber (grams): 5
Total fruit and vegetable (servings): 3½, including 1 serving
  of cruciferous vegetable

For prostate protection: *For minimal fat, use ¼ instead of ½ teaspoon canola oil.*

BROCCOLI-MUSHROOM STIR-FRY WITH TOFU

In this recipe we use fresh shiitake mushrooms. Don't be put off by the price and don't skimp on them. They make the dish! Since the flavor is so rich, four small mushrooms flavor the whole dish. Because so little oil is used to sauté the broccoli and cauliflower, make sure they are in small pieces.

YIELD: 2 SERVINGS
PREPARATION TIME: 10 MINUTES
COOKING TIME: 15 MINUTES

INGREDIENTS:
¼ teaspoon canola oil
1 cup broccoli florets (grape-size pieces)
2 cloves roasted garlic, minced
18 snow peas
4 small shiitake mushrooms, chopped
4 medium green onions, chopped
½ cup sliced water chestnuts
6 drops chili oil
6 drops tamari soy sauce
1 teaspoon sherry vinegar
1 teaspoon freshly grated ginger
4 ounces firm tofu, in irregular-shaped pieces
2 cups cooked brown rice (page 178)

1. In a large skillet or wok, heat canola oil over medium heat. Add broccoli and garlic; cook about 5 minutes, stirring constantly.
2. Add snow peas, mushrooms, green onions, and water chestnuts. Cook about 5 minutes longer, stirring constantly.
3. Add chili oil, soy sauce, sherry vinegar, and ginger; gently mix into vegetables.
4. Add tofu. Stir gently. Continue cooking 2 to 3 minutes, just to heat tofu.
5. Serve over brown rice.

Estimated nutrients per serving:
Calories: 300
Total protein (grams): 12
Soy protein (grams): 4
Total carbohydrate (grams): 58
Total fat (grams): 3.5

Total fiber (grams): 8

Total fruit and vegetable (servings): 2, including 1 serving of cruciferous vegetable

For prostate protection: *To increase lycopene, add 1 medium tomato, chopped, in step 2.*

SWEET AND SOUR TOFU

Sweet and sour dishes are always popular. In this recipe, pineapple contributes the sweetness and vinegar the sourness.

YIELD: 2 SERVINGS

PREPARATION TIME: 20 MINUTES

COOKING TIME: 15 MINUTES

INGREDIENTS:
   1½ tablespoons cornstarch
   ½ cup rice vinegar
   ½ cup pineapple juice concentrate
   ½ teaspoon tamari soy sauce
   2 tablespoons brown sugar
   ½ cup canned pineapple chunks
   5 ounces extra-firm tofu, cubed
   ½ teaspoon canola oil
   ½ medium onion, cut in large chunks
   ½ medium sweet red pepper, stems, seeds, and membranes
      removed; cut in large chunks
   1 cup broccoli florets
   2 cups cooked brown rice (page 178)

1. Place cornstarch in a small saucepan. Add half of the rice vinegar and stir until smooth. Add the remaining rice vinegar, pineapple juice concentrate, soy sauce, and brown sugar.
2. Cook over medium heat until mixture thickens. Add pineapple and tofu. Set aside.
3. In a large skillet, heat canola oil over medium heat; add onion. Cook for 5 minutes, until soft.

4. Add red pepper and broccoli; continue to cook for 3 to 5 minutes longer.
5. Pour the sauce mixture over the vegetables; stir gently while re-heating.
6. Serve over brown rice.

Estimated nutrients per serving:
Calories: 410
Total protein (grams): 12
Soy protein (grams): 5
Total carbohydrate (grams): 84
Total fat (grams): 4
Total fiber (grams): 7
Total fruit and vegetable (servings): 3½, including 1 serving of cruciferous vegetable

For prostate protection: *For minimal fat, use ¼ instead of ½ teaspoon canola oil.*

VEGETABLES AND TOFU WITH NOODLES

Barbara's Aussie friend Helen called this an over-the-top vegetable dish because it is so chock-full of vegetables providing a variety of colors and textures.

YIELD: 2 SERVINGS
PREPARATION TIME: 20 MINUTES
COOKING TIME: 10 MINUTES

INGREDIENTS:
2 medium dried black mushrooms
¾ cup hot water
1 tablespoon hoisin sauce
1½ teaspoons rice wine vinegar
6 drops chili oil
6 drops sesame oil
1 teaspoon freshly grated ginger

⅓ cup water
½ teaspoon canola oil
½ cup cauliflower florets (grape-size pieces)
½ cup broccoli florets (grape-size pieces)
½ small red onion, cut in chunks
½ cup chopped bok choy
¼ medium sweet red pepper, cut in chunks
¼ cup sliced water chestnuts
¼ cup sliced bamboo shoots
4 ounces extra-firm tofu, cubed
2 cups cooked rice noodles
2 large sprigs cilantro

1. Rinse mushrooms under cold water. In a small bowl soak mushrooms in the ¾ cup hot water for 20 minutes or until soft. Drain; slice mushrooms. Set aside.
2. In another small bowl combine hoisin sauce, vinegar, chili and sesame oils, ginger, and the ⅓ cup water. Set aside.
3. In a medium skillet or wok, heat canola oil over medium-high heat. Add cauliflower, broccoli, and onion; cook for 5 minutes, stirring constantly.
4. Add bok choy and red pepper; continue to cook for 3 minutes.
5. Add reserved mushrooms to skillet. Stir in water chestnuts, bamboo shoots, and sauce mixture.
6. Add tofu; stir gently to combine.
7. Serve over rice noodles. Garnish with cilantro.

Estimated nutrients per serving:
Calories: 220
Total protein (grams): 8
Soy protein (grams): 4
Total carbohydrate (grams): 42
Total fat (grams): 2.5
Total fiber (grams): 4
Total fruit and vegetable (servings): 2½, including 1½ servings of cruciferous vegetable

For prostate protection: For minimal fat, use ¼ instead of ½ teaspoon canola oil.

FRESH SOYBEANS AND VEGETABLES WITH BLACK BEAN SAUCE

Black bean sauce is made from fermented black beans and has a rich pungent flavor. It is used to season many Asian dishes and provides the complementary background flavor for this dish.

YIELD: 2 SERVINGS

PREPARATION TIME: 15 MINUTES

COOKING TIME: 5 MINUTES

INGREDIENTS:

1 tablespoon cornstarch
1 cup water
1 tablespoon dry sherry
½ tablespoon tamari soy sauce
Pinch sugar
1 tablespoon black bean sauce
1 teaspoon canola oil
3 medium green onions, chopped
4 cloves roasted garlic, crushed
1 cup cauliflower florets (grape-size pieces)
1 cup sweet red pepper strips
½ cup 1-inch pieces Chinese long beans or other green beans
1 cup fresh green soybeans
2 cups cooked brown rice (page 178)

1. In a small bowl, mix cornstarch with ¼ cup of the water to a smooth paste. Add remaining water, sherry, soy sauce, sugar, and black bean sauce. Stir to combine; set aside.
2. In a medium nonstick skillet or wok, heat canola oil over medium-high heat; add green onions, garlic, cauliflower, sweet red pepper, and green beans. Cook for 2 minutes, stirring constantly. Add soybeans; stir to mix.
3. Add cornstarch mixture; stir constantly until sauce comes to a boil.
4. Serve over brown rice.

Estimated nutrients per serving:
Calories: 430
Total protein (grams): 19

Soy protein (grams): 11
Total carbohydrate (grams): 68
Total fat (grams): 10
Total fiber (grams): 11
Total fruit and vegetable (servings): 4, including 1 serving of cruciferous vegetable

For prostate protection: *For minimal fat, use ½ instead of 1 teaspoon canola oil.*

CAULIFLOWER AND CARROT CURRY WITH TOFU

A curry is a blend of spices. There are many variations of curry that reflect regional or family preferences. This recipe uses a mixture of fresh ginger, cumin, coriander, and turmeric. Be adventurous and try your own combination of spices, or use one of the commercial curry powder blends available in place of the spices in this recipe.

The turmeric gives this dish a pretty yellow color. And the mix of ginger, cumin, coriander, and turmeric gives the meal an exotic flavor.

YIELD: 2 SERVINGS
PREPARATION TIME: 15 MINUTES
COOKING TIME: 15 MINUTES

INGREDIENTS:
  2 *tablespoons cornstarch*
  1¾ *cups water*
  ½ *teaspoon canola oil*
  ¼ *medium onion, chopped*
  2 *cloves roasted garlic, minced*
  ½ *tablespoon freshly grated ginger*
  1 *teaspoon cumin powder*
  1 *teaspoon dried coriander leaf*
  ⅛ *teaspoon turmeric*
  1 *cup small cauliflower florets*
  1 *small carrot, thinly sliced*
  1 *cup sliced green beans*
  1 *small tomato, chopped*

4 ounces extra-firm tofu, cubed
2 cups cooked brown rice (page 178)
1 tablespoon chopped fresh cilantro

1. In a small bowl, mix cornstarch with ¼ cup of the water to a smooth paste. Add remaining water; stir to combine. Set aside.
2. In a medium skillet or wok, heat canola oil over medium-high heat. Add onion and garlic. Cook for 3 minutes.
3. Stir in ginger, cumin, coriander, and turmeric. Add cauliflower, carrot, and green beans. Cook for 4 minutes.
4. Gently stir in tomato and cook for 3 minutes to heat tomato.
5. Pour cornstarch mixture over the vegetables. Bring to a boil, stirring constantly.
6. Add tofu; stir gently and cook for 1 minute to warm the tofu.
7. Serve over brown rice and garnish with fresh cilantro.

Estimated nutrients per serving:
Calories: 330
Total protein (grams): 12
Soy protein (grams): 4
Total carbohydrate (grams): 65
Total fat (grams): 4
Total fiber (grams): 8
Total fruit and vegetable (servings): 3, including 1 serving of cruciferous vegetable

For prostate protection: *For minimal fat, use ¼ instead of ½ teaspoon canola oil.*

SWEET AND SOUR BOK CHOY AND TEMPEH

Bok choy is a variety of Chinese cabbage also known as Chinese chard. We prefer to use the young, tender baby bok choy.

YIELD: 2 SERVINGS
PREPARATION TIME: 15 MINUTES
COOKING TIME: 10 MINUTES

INGREDIENTS:

2 tablespoons cornstarch
1 cup pineapple juice
1 tablespoon sherry
4 teaspoons tamari soy sauce
2 tablespoons white vinegar
8 drops chili oil
½ teaspoon canola oil
1 medium carrot, sliced
½ medium green pepper, sliced
½ medium red onion, chopped
1 cup chopped baby bok choy
4 ounces tempeh, cubed
½ cup pineapple chunks
1 tablespoon freshly grated ginger
2 cups cooked brown rice (page 178)

1. In a small bowl, combine cornstarch with ¼ cup of the pineapple juice to make a smooth paste. Add remaining pineapple juice, sherry, soy sauce, vinegar, and chili oil. Stir to combine; set aside.
2. In a medium skillet or wok, heat canola oil over medium heat; add carrot, green pepper, and onion. Cook for 5 minutes, stirring constantly.
3. Add cornstarch mixture; stir constantly until sauce comes to a boil.
4. Add bok choy, tempeh, pineapple, and ginger; stir gently to combine and heat for 2 minutes.
5. Serve over brown rice.

Estimated nutrients per serving:
Calories: 500
Total protein (grams): 18
Soy protein (grams): 11
Total carbohydrate (grams): 92
Total fat (grams): 8
Total fiber (grams): 12
Total fruit and vegetable (servings): 2½, including 1 serving of cruciferous vegetable

For prostate protection: For minimal fat, use ¼ instead of ½ teaspoon canola oil.

GRILLED FRESH TUNA

When we were working on this book, Rita's neighbor opened a fish market in Oakland, called Young Tuna Seafood Company, named after the mascot in the Samoan village where the owner spent his childhood. The fresh tuna at Young Tuna looked especially good and inspired this recipe.

The cooked tuna has the texture and flavor of a pork chop, and that makes it a perfect choice for when you're craving meat.

YIELD: 2 SERVINGS

PREPARATION TIME: 5 MINUTES, PLUS 1 HOUR OF
    STANDING TIME

COOKING TIME: 10 MINUTES

INGREDIENTS:

¼ cup fish sauce
Juice of 2 limes
2 teaspoons freshly grated ginger
2 (4-ounce) pieces fresh tuna
2 wedges fresh lime
2 sprigs cilantro

1. In a flat dish large enough to hold the tuna in a single layer, combine the fish sauce, lime juice, and ginger. Add fish; turn fish over a few times to cover both sides well. Cover and marinate for 1 hour.
2. Preheat broiler. Place tuna on a broiler pan; place in preheated oven and broil for 4 minutes on each side or until done.
3. Serve garnished with lime wedges and cilantro.

Estimated nutrients per serving:

Calories: 160
Total protein (grams): 26
Soy protein (grams): 0
Total carbohydrate (grams): 0
Total fat (grams): 6
Total fiber (grams): 0
Total fruit and vegetable (servings): none

For prostate protection: *To eliminate animal products, use 4 ounces baked tofu instead of tuna.*

RICE NOODLES WITH VEGETABLES AND TOFU IN BLACK BEAN SAUCE

The inspiration for this recipe came from a visit to a local farmers market. We envisioned the vibrant colors of the produce contrasting with the white tofu.

YIELD: 2 SERVINGS

PREPARATION TIME: 20 MINUTES

COOKING TIME: 15 MINUTES

INGREDIENTS:
  1 tablespoon cornstarch
  2 tablespoons cold water
  ¾ cup vegetable stock, homemade (page 88) or canned
  ½ tablespoon black bean sauce
  1 teaspoon canola oil
  ¼ medium onion, cut in large chunks
  ¼ cup diagonally sliced carrot
  ½ cup diagonally sliced green beans
  ½ cup small broccoli florets
  ½ cup sliced baby bok choy stems and leaves
  3 small shiitake mushrooms, sliced
  ¼ medium sweet red pepper, cut in ½-inch squares
  3½ ounces extra-firm tofu, cut in ½-inch cubes
  2 cups cooked rice noodles

1. In a small bowl, mix cornstarch with water to a smooth paste. Add stock and black bean sauce. Stir to combine. Set aside.
2. In a medium skillet or wok, heat oil over medium-high heat. Add onion; cook for 3 minutes or until soft but not brown.
3. Add carrot; cook for another 3 minutes.
4. Add green beans, broccoli, and bok choy. Cook for 2 minutes.

5. Add mushrooms and red pepper. Cook for 2 minutes.
6. Pour cornstarch mixture over vegetables. Bring to a boil, stirring constantly.
7. Add tofu. Stir gently to mix. Continue cooking for another 2 minutes to heat the tofu.
8. Serve over rice noodles.

Estimated nutrients per serving:
Calories: 230
Total protein (grams): 7
Soy protein (grams): 4
Total carbohydrate (grams): 45
Total fat (grams): 3
Total fiber (grams): 4
Total fruit and vegetable (servings): 2½, including 1 serving of cruciferous vegetable

For prostate protection: *For minimal fat, use ½ instead of 1 teaspoon canola oil.*

CURRIED SOYBEANS AND BROCCOLI

When developing this recipe, we decided to marry the complexity of flavors of the spices with broccoli and soybeans. The cilantro and lemon wedge used as a garnish provide a tantalizing contrast.

YIELD: 2 SERVINGS
PREPARATION TIME: 15 MINUTES
COOKING TIME: 30 MINUTES

INGREDIENTS:
¼ teaspoon canola oil
¼ medium onion, chopped
1 cup small broccoli florets
1 small Granny Smith apple, peeled and chopped
¼ teaspoon freshly grated ginger
½ teaspoon ground cumin
¼ teaspoon ground cardamom
1 teaspoon ground coriander, divided

⅛ teaspoon ground turmeric
⅛ teaspoon ground cinnamon
⅛ teaspoon red pepper flakes
1 cup water
1 medium tomato, chopped
1 cup cooked mature soybeans (page 181) or canned soybeans
¼ cup plain nonfat yogurt
2 cups cooked brown rice (page 178)
10 medium cilantro leaves, coarsely chopped
2 small lemon wedges

1. In a large saucepan, heat the oil over medium-high heat. Add onion; cook 3 minutes, until brown, stirring constantly.
2. Add broccoli and apple. Continue cooking for 3 minutes.
3. Add ginger, cumin, cardamom, ½ teaspoon coriander, turmeric, cinnamon, and pepper flakes. Reduce heat to low; cook for 1 minute, stirring constantly.
4. Add water. Bring to a boil. Reduce heat, cover, and simmer for 15 minutes. Stir in tomato and soybeans; cook for 5 minutes longer.
5. Add yogurt and ½ teaspoon ground coriander. Stir gently to combine. Do not boil.
6. Serve over brown rice; sprinkle with cilantro and garnish with lemon wedges.

Estimated nutrients per serving:
Calories: 420
Total protein (grams): 20
Soy protein (grams): 11
Total carbohydrate (grams): 71
Total fat (grams): 9
Total fiber (grams): 10
Total fruit and vegetable (servings): 2, including 1 serving of cruciferous vegetable

For prostate protection: *To eliminate animal products, omit nonfat yogurt.*

TOFU KEBOBS

This is great for grilling on the barbecue in the summertime. It's ideal to put together when friends drop by unexpectedly because you'll probably have the ingredients on hand and it requires so little time to prepare and cook. Don't be alarmed by the tablespoon of oil used in the marinade — most of it drips off during cooking.

YIELD: 2 SERVINGS
PREPARATION TIME: 10 MINUTES
COOKING TIME: 10 MINUTES

INGREDIENTS:

1 tablespoon sesame oil
1 tablespoon tamari soy sauce
1 teaspoon rice vinegar
2 drops chili oil
½ teaspoon honey
1 (7-ounce) package teriyaki baked tofu, cubed
1 medium sweet red pepper, stem, seeds, and membranes removed;
   cut in large chunks
1 cup pineapple chunks, drained
2 cups cooked brown rice (page 178)

1. In a small teacup or bowl, combine sesame oil, soy sauce, vinegar, chili oil, and honey.
2. Thread tofu, red pepper, and pineapple alternately on skewers. Brush with soy sauce mixture.
3. Place skewers on broiler pan. Place pan under preheated broiler and broil for 2 minutes.
4. Brush again with mixture. Turn over; broil for 2 more minutes.
5. Remove from skewers and serve over rice.

Estimated nutrients per serving:

Calories: 310
Total protein (grams): 13
Soy protein (grams): 7
Total carbohydrate (grams): 60
Total fat (grams): 3.5
Total fiber (grams): 7
Total fruit and vegetable (servings): 2

For prostate protection: *For minimal dietary fat, use marinade sparingly.*

FISH WITH CARROT AND BROCCOLI IN PLUM SAUCE

In this delicious and filling dish, the flavor combination of the plum sauce and prepared black soybeans is superb.

YIELD: 2 SERVINGS
PREPARATION TIME: 10 MINUTES
COOKING TIME: 15 MINUTES

INGREDIENTS:

2 tablespoons cornstarch
½ cup water
2 tablespoons plum sauce
2 teaspoons canola oil
1 large green onion, chopped
1 medium carrot, sliced diagonally
1 cup small broccoli florets
1 teaspoon freshly grated ginger
6 ounces halibut, cubed
1 (6.35-ounce) can prepared black soybeans; remove the seaweed
    (called tangle) and chestnuts, then rinse
1 teaspoon fresh lemon juice
2 cups cooked brown rice (page 178)

1. In a small bowl, mix cornstarch with ¼ cup of the water to a smooth paste. Add remaining water and plum sauce. Stir to combine; set aside.
2. In a medium skillet or wok, heat oil over medium-high heat. Add green onion, carrot, broccoli, and ginger. Cook for 5 minutes, stirring constantly.
3. Add cornstarch mixture. Bring to a boil, stirring constantly. Reduce heat; add fish and cook for 5 to 7 minutes, until fish is cooked through. Add soybeans and cook for 1 minute longer. Gently stir in the lemon juice.
4. Serve over rice.

Estimated nutrients per serving:
Calories: 480
Total protein (grams): 30

Soy protein (grams): 7
Total carbohydrate (grams): 66
Total fat (grams): 11
Total fiber (grams): 9
Total fruit and vegetable (servings): 2, including 1 serving of cruciferous vegetable

For prostate protection: *This recipe cannot be modified to meet the prostate cancer recommendations.*

SWEET AND SOUR CHICKEN

This easy-to-prepare recipe is a favorite of Rita's family. When her schedule is unusually busy, she prepares this ahead of time to have ready to pop into the oven when she comes home from work. The pineapple keeps the baked chicken moist and adds sweetness. The contrast between the cooked meat and the fruit is a delightful surprise to the palate.

YIELD: 4 SERVINGS
PREPARATION TIME: 10 MINUTES
COOKING TIME: 50 MINUTES

INGREDIENTS:
  1 (8-ounce) can crushed pineapple (in its own juice)
  1½ tablespoons cornstarch
  1 cup water
  2 teaspoons tamari soy sauce
  1 teaspoon rice vinegar
  ½ teaspoon freshly grated ginger
  4 medium boneless, skinless chicken breast halves
  2 cups cooked brown rice (page 178)

Preheat oven to 400 degrees.
  1. Drain pineapple, reserving juice.
  2. In a small saucepan, combine cornstarch with ¼ cup of the water to make a smooth paste. Add remaining water, soy sauce, vinegar, ginger, and reserved pineapple juice. Cook over medium-high heat, stirring gently and constantly, until mixture comes to a boil and is thickened.

3. Place chicken breasts in a single layer in a shallow baking dish. Pour mixture over chicken, cover, and place in preheated oven for 30 minutes, basting several times.
4. Spoon pineapple over the chicken. Bake uncovered for an additional 15 minutes.
5. Serve over brown rice.

Estimated nutrients per serving:
Calories: 380
Total protein (grams): 32
Soy protein (grams): 0
Total carbohydrate (grams): 49
Total fat (grams): 6
Total fiber (grams): 4
Total fruit and vegetable (servings): 1

For prostate protection: *This recipe cannot be modified to meet the prostate cancer recommendations.*

NOODLES WITH CELERY, CARROT, AND BROCCOLI

This combination of hearty vegetables and baked tofu served with noodles is a wonderful meal to have at the end of a busy day. Because it goes together so quickly, you can take more time to relax and enjoy the meal.

YIELD: 2 SERVINGS
PREPARATION TIME: 15 MINUTES
COOKING TIME: 5 MINUTES

INGREDIENTS:
1 tablespoon cornstarch
1 cup vegetable stock, homemade (page 88) or canned
¼ teaspoon freshly grated ginger
6 drops chili oil
4 ounces Asian-style vermicelli noodles
½ teaspoon canola oil

3 cloves roasted garlic, minced
1 medium green onion, sliced
1 stalk celery, trimmed and thinly sliced on the diagonal
1 small carrot, thinly sliced on the diagonal
1 cup small broccoli florets
¼ cup bamboo shoots
3½ ounces savory baked tofu, cubed
1 tablespoon chopped peanuts
2 sprigs cilantro

1. In a small bowl, combine cornstarch with 2 tablespoons of the stock to make a smooth paste. Add remaining stock, ginger, and chili oil. Stir to combine; set aside.
2. Cook noodles according to package directions. Keep warm.
3. In a medium skillet or wok, heat canola oil over medium-high heat; add garlic, onion, celery, carrot, and broccoli. Cook for 3 minutes, stirring constantly. Add bamboo shoots and stir to combine.
4. Add cornstarch mixture; stir constantly until sauce comes to a boil. Stir in tofu.
5. Serve over noodles. Sprinkle with peanuts and garnish with cilantro.

Estimated nutrients per serving:
Calories: 300
Total protein (grams): 14
Soy protein (grams): 4
Total carbohydrate (grams): 49
Total fat (grams): 6
Total fiber (grams): 5
Total fruit and vegetable (servings): 2, including 1 serving of cruciferous vegetable

For prostate protection: For minimal fat, use ¼ instead of ½ teaspoon canola oil; omit peanuts.

NEW AMERICAN

BEAN AND BROCCOLI BURRITO
WITH TOMATO-CORN SALSA

Because so little oil is used to sauté the broccoli, make sure the broccoli is in small (grape-size) pieces. The filling and salsa can be prepared in advance. Reheat filling before assembling burritos.

YIELD: 2 SERVINGS, 1 BURRITO EACH
PREPARATION TIME: 30 MINUTES
COOKING TIME: NONE

INGREDIENTS:

¼ teaspoon canola oil
⅔ cup broccoli florets (grape-size pieces)
4 medium green onions, chopped
⅔ cup cooked brown rice (page 178)
⅔ cup canned black beans, drained, not rinsed
½ cup chopped tomato
¼ cup white corn, fresh or frozen
2 tablespoons chopped cilantro
2 (10-inch) flour tortillas
2 tablespoons grated low-fat cheddar cheese
Sprinkle red chili powder, if desired

1. Heat oil over medium heat in a nonstick pan; add broccoli and green onions. Stir constantly, about 3 to 5 minutes, until vegetables are soft.
2. Add brown rice and black beans; cook until mixture is hot, stirring gently.
3. Make salsa by mixing tomato, corn, and cilantro in a small bowl.
4. Soften tortillas by placing in a hot skillet for a few seconds.
5. Spread rice and bean mixture along center of tortilla; sprinkle cheese over mixture. Top with salsa. Add chili powder if desired.
6. Fold opposite sides of tortilla over about 1 inch of filling, then roll the tortilla over the filling.

Estimated nutrients per serving:
Calories: 440
Total protein (grams): 17
Soy protein (grams): 0
Total carbohydrate (grams): 70
Total fat (grams): 8
Total fiber (grams): 9
Total fruit and vegetable (servings): 1½, including 1 serving
 of cruciferous vegetable

For prostate protection: *To eliminate animal products, omit low-fat cheese.*

BAKED BEANS

Baked beans are as American as the Fourth of July and are often a staple at pot lucks, picnics, and barbecues. This is an adaptation of a favorite family recipe for picnics across the country. It's great with Healthy Coleslaw, page 211.

YIELD: 6 SERVINGS
PREPARATION TIME: 20 MINUTES
COOKING TIME: 40 MINUTES

INGREDIENTS:
 1 teaspoon olive oil
 1 large onion, chopped
 4 cloves roasted garlic, minced
 1 (15-ounce) can soybeans, drained, not rinsed; or 2 cups cooked
  mature soybeans (page 181)
 1 (15-ounce) can baby lima beans, drained, not rinsed
 1 (15-ounce) can red kidney beans, drained, not rinsed
 ¼ cup light brown sugar
 1½ tablespoons molasses
 ¾ cup catsup
 3 tablespoons cider vinegar
 ¼ cup water
 ¾ teaspoon prepared mustard
 ½ teaspoon salt

Preheat oven to 350 degrees.

1. In a medium skillet, heat olive oil over medium-high heat. Add onion and garlic and cook for 15 minutes, until onion is deep golden.
2. Meanwhile, combine all the beans in a 2½-quart casserole dish.
3. In a small bowl, mix brown sugar, molasses, catsup, vinegar, water, mustard and salt; add to beans.
4. Add onion-garlic mixture; stir gently.
5. Bake in preheated oven for 40 minutes.

Estimated nutrients per serving:

Calories: 395
Total protein (grams): 15
Soy protein (grams): 12
Total carbohydrate (grams): 62
Total fat (grams): 8
Total fiber (grams): 15
Total fruit and vegetable (servings): none

For prostate protection: *For minimal fat, use ½ instead of 1 teaspoon olive oil.*

MACARONI AND CHEESE

Kids of all ages love macaroni and cheese. The creamy texture of this dish comes in part from the soy protein powder. This recipe tastes best with a very sharp reduced-fat cheddar cheese.

YIELD: 2 SERVINGS
PREPARATION TIME: 20 MINUTES
COOKING TIME: 20 MINUTES

INGREDIENTS:

2 quarts water
¼ teaspoon salt
1 cup macaroni
1 tablespoon cornstarch
2 tablespoons packed soy protein powder

¼ *teaspoon salt*
1 *cup nonfat soy milk*
½ *cup reduced-fat cheddar cheese*
⅛ *teaspoon pepper*
Pinch nutmeg

Preheat oven to 350 degrees.
1. Bring water and ¼ teaspoon salt to a boil. Add macaroni and cook for 12 to 15 minutes, until tender. Drain.
2. Meanwhile, in a small saucepan, thoroughly mix the cornstarch, soy protein powder, and ¼ teaspoon salt.
3. Gradually stir in ¼ cup of the soy milk until mixture is smooth.
4. Add remaining soy milk and stir until well blended.
5. Cook over medium heat; stirring constantly, until thickened.
6. Remove from heat; stir in cheese, pepper, and nutmeg.
7. Stir in macaroni. Pour into 1-quart casserole; cover and bake in preheated oven for 20 minutes.

Estimated nutrients per serving:
Calories: 410
Total protein (grams): 26
Soy protein (grams): 11
Total carbohydrate (grams): 66
Total fat (grams): 3.5
Total fiber (grams): 4
Total fruit and vegetable (servings): none

For prostate protection: *This recipe cannot be modified to meet the prostate cancer recommendations.*

GRILLED SWORDFISH WITH ROASTED CORN AND RED PEPPER SALSA

Swordfish has a mild flavor that appeals to many people. The swordfish can be cooked over an outdoor grill. The Roasted Corn and Red Pepper Salsa provides a Southwestern flair and looks elegant on the swordfish. The wonderful flavors of the salsa complement the mild-tasting swordfish. Salmon or trout may be substituted for the swordfish.

YIELD: 2 SERVINGS

PREPARATION TIME: 25 MINUTES

COOKING TIME: 10 MINUTES

INGREDIENTS:

1 ear sweet corn

½ medium sweet red pepper

¼ teaspoon olive oil

2 (4-ounce) portions swordfish

1½ teaspoons chopped cilantro

⅛ teaspoon salt

Preheat oven to 400 degrees.

1. Remove husks and silk from corn. Rinse corn and cut kernels from cob. Place on foil-lined cookie sheet.
2. Remove stem, seeds, and membranes from pepper. Rinse pepper; place on cookie sheet with corn.
3. Roast corn and pepper in oven for 15 minutes. Remove from oven; let cool. Preheat broiler.
4. Spread the olive oil over both sides of each portion of fish. Place on grilling rack; broil for 5 minutes on each side, or until fish flakes easily with a fork.
5. Meanwhile, peel loose skin from pepper, dice finely. Combine pepper, corn, cilantro, and salt. Stir lightly to mix.
6. Serve fish topped with salsa.

Estimated nutrients per serving:

Calories: 200

Total protein (grams): 21

Soy protein (grams): 0

Total carbohydrate (grams): 14

Total fat (grams): 6

Total fiber (grams): 2

Total fruit and vegetable (servings): 1

For prostate protection:

■ *To increase lycopene, add ½ cup chopped tomato to the salsa.*

■ *To eliminate animal products, use 2- to 3-ounce portions of savory baked tofu instead of the swordfish; broil for 3 minutes on each side.*

STUFFED RED PEPPER

The red pepper, green broccoli, and black beans make this dish visually appealing in addition to being good to eat! Red peppers are a great source of the antioxidants beta-carotene and vitamin C.

YIELD: 2 SERVINGS
PREPARATION TIME: 15 MINUTES
COOKING TIME: 40 MINUTES

INGREDIENTS:

¾ cup small broccoli florets
2 tablespoons chopped green onion
½ cup cooked brown rice (page 178)
½ cup cooked wild rice (page 179)
¼ cup canned black beans
1 tablespoon raisins
2 tablespoons tomato sauce
⅛ teaspoon salt
1 large evenly shaped sweet red pepper
2 tablespoons grated low-fat cheddar cheese

Preheat oven to 375 degrees.

1. Blanch broccoli and green onion together.
2. Mix all ingredients except red pepper and cheese.
3. Cut pepper in half lengthwise; remove stem, seeds, and membranes; rinse pepper.
4. Put half of the vegetable-rice mixture in each pepper half.
5. Place in an ovenproof dish; cover with foil. Bake for 35 minutes.
6. Remove from oven; top each pepper half with 1 tablespoon grated cheese. Return to oven, uncovered, for about 2 minutes, until cheese is melted.

Estimated nutrients per serving:

Calories: 200
Total protein (grams): 10
Soy protein (grams): 0
Total carbohydrate (grams): 40
Total fat (grams): 1.5
Total fiber (grams): 7

Total fruit and vegetable (servings): 2, including 1 serving of cruciferous vegetable

For prostate protection: *To eliminate animal products, top with toasted whole wheat bread crumbs instead of low-fat cheese.*

COTTAGE PIE

ottage Pie is a dish that the English traditionally make on Monday to use the leftovers from weekend meals. This version surprises you with a sweet potato crust instead of the predictable white potato crust. It can go together quickly with cooked lentils and brown rice. Other leftover vegetables, legumes, or grains can be substituted for those in the recipe.

YIELD: 4 SERVINGS
PREPARATION TIME: 30 MINUTES, PLUS 1 HOUR TO COOK SWEET POTATOES
COOKING TIME: 30 MINUTES

INGREDIENTS:
   2 large sweet potatoes
   ¼ medium onion
   1 cup shredded green cabbage
   1 large carrot, cut in chunks
   1 medium rutabaga, cut in ½-inch cubes
   1 cup cooked lentils (page 179)
   1 cup cooked brown rice (page 178)
   1 cup cooked mature soybeans (page 181)
   2 cups vegetable gravy (page 89)
   2 tablespoons chopped parsley
   1 teaspoon salt
   ½ teaspoon pepper

Preheat oven to 375 degrees.
   1. Scrub sweet potatoes; cut into quarters.
   2. Place onion and sweet potato on a cookie sheet lined with foil; put in preheated oven.

3. Bake for approximately 1 hour, until sweet potato is very soft; remove from oven and let cool.
4. Meanwhile, blanch cabbage. Blanch carrot and rutabaga together.
5. Chop onion and combine with all other ingredients, except the sweet potato.
6. Pour into 1½-quart casserole dish.
7. Peel and mash sweet potatoes. Spoon over filling; spread evenly with a fork.
8. Bake uncovered for 30 minutes.

Estimated nutrients per serving:
Calories: 340
Total protein (grams): 16
Soy protein (grams): 7
Total carbohydrate (grams): 62
Total fat (grams): 5
Total fiber (grams): 13
Total fruit and vegetable (servings): 2½, including 1 serving of cruciferous vegetable

For prostate protection: *You can use this recipe as is.*

GRILLED SALMON WITH SESAME AND LIME

The tangy aromatic flavors of sesame and lime provide a wonderful contrast to the richness of the salmon.

Brushing the salmon with a little oil before broiling gives it a crispy surface. The light tartar sauce goes well with the rich fish, and the crunchy gherkin pieces add a wonderful texture. Also, the subtle contrast in flavors is delicious — rich salmon, mild yogurt, sweet gherkin, and slightly sour capers. One taste judge commented that this is excellent and so easy to make. He would happily serve it at a dinner party.

YIELD: 2 SERVINGS

PREPARATION TIME: 5 MINUTES

COOKING TIME: 10 TO 16 MINUTES

INGREDIENTS:
½ teaspoon olive oil
2 drops sesame oil
2 (4-ounce) salmon fillets
2 wedges lime

Tartar sauce:
2 tablespoons silken tofu
2 tablespoons plain nonfat yogurt
½ teaspoon extra-virgin olive oil
½ medium sweet gherkin pickle, finely chopped
1 teaspoon capers, minced
¼ teaspoon fresh lemon juice

Preheat broiler.
1. Combine oils; brush over both sides of salmon fillets.
2. Put salmon on a broiler pan, place in preheated oven, and broil for 5 to 8 minutes on each side, depending on thickness of fillet.
3. Meanwhile, make tartar sauce by blending tofu, yogurt, and olive oil until smooth. Add pickle, capers, and lemon juice; combine.
4. Serve fish with lime wedges and tartar sauce.

Estimated nutrients per serving:
Calories: 210
Total protein (grams): 26
Soy protein (grams): 1
Total carbohydrate (grams): 4
Total fat (grams): 9
Total fiber (grams): 0
Total fruit and vegetable (servings): none

For prostate protection: *This recipe cannot be modified to meet the prostate cancer recommendations.*

SPAGHETTI WITH TOMATO-TEMPEH SAUCE

Because spaghetti with meat sauce is a mainstay of the American diet, we developed this recipe using whole wheat noodles and a tomato-tempeh sauce. The tempeh is quite filling, so you really feel that you've had a complete, satisfying meal. Like any popular tomato sauce, the flavors blend over time to give a sauce with more interesting character. This sauce keeps well, so prepare a large amount and refrigerate or freeze it for a quick meal later. One of the judges was particularly impressed. She said, "This is absolutely DELICIOUS! It's definitely one of my favorite recipes in the book. Although it's in the New American section, the olives, garlic, and oregano give it a Mediterranean flavor."

YIELD: 2 SERVINGS

PREPARATION TIME: 15 MINUTES

COOKING TIME: 20 MINUTES FOR SAUCE,
   15 MINUTES FOR PASTA

INGREDIENTS:
For sauce:
½ large green bell pepper
½ medium onion, chopped
4 large mushrooms, sliced
1 clove roasted garlic, minced
4 ounces soy tempeh, crumbled
6 large Italian olives, sliced
2 cups tomato sauce
½ teaspoon oregano
¼ teaspoon pepper
¼ teaspoon salt

For spaghetti:
2 quarts water
¼ teaspoon salt
4 ounces whole wheat spaghetti
2 tablespoons freshly grated Parmesan cheese

1. Remove stem, seeds, and membranes from green pepper; cut in half lengthwise and slice across.
2. Put green pepper, onion, mushrooms, and garlic in a preheated non-stick saucepan; sauté for about 10 minutes, until vegetables are soft.
3. Add tempeh, olives, tomato sauce, oregano, pepper, and salt; cook over medium heat for 10 minutes, until all ingredients are heated through. Keep warm.

4. To cook the spaghetti, bring water to a boil; add salt. Add spaghetti and cook for 12 to 15 minutes, until tender.

5. Drain spaghetti. Divide between 2 plates or pasta bowls.

6. Top with sauce and sprinkle with Parmesan cheese.

Estimated nutrients per serving:
Calories: 460
Total protein (grams): 25
Soy protein (grams): 11
Total carbohydrate (grams): 77
Total fat (grams): 9
Total fiber (grams): 13
Total fruit and vegetable (servings): 3

For prostate protection: *To eliminate animal products, sprinkle with chopped Italian parsley instead of Parmesan cheese.*

ENGLISH CHICKEN-MUSHROOM CASSEROLE

Mushroom broth intensifies the mushroom flavor of this dish. Look for it in fancy food stores. If you can't find mushroom broth, you can substitute vegetable broth.

YIELD: 2 SERVINGS
PREPARATION TIME: 30 MINUTES
COOKING TIME: 30 MINUTES

INGREDIENTS:
1 cup bulgur (cracked wheat)
¾ cup mushroom broth
½ teaspoon olive oil
½ medium onion, chopped
2 cloves roasted garlic, minced
4 medium mushrooms, sliced
½ medium rutabaga, diced in ¼-inch pieces
½ cup frozen peas
½ teaspoon olive oil
2 (3-ounce) skinless, boneless chicken breasts, cut in 1-inch pieces

½ *cup mushroom broth*
¼ *teaspoon thyme*

Preheat oven to 350 degrees.
1. Place bulgur in 1½-quart casserole dish. Bring the ¾ cup broth to a boil and pour over bulgur. Set aside.
2. Heat ½ teaspoon olive oil in a medium skillet over medium heat; add onion and garlic. Cook for 10 minutes, until onion is golden.
3. Add mushrooms and continue to cook 5 minutes longer. Stir in rutabaga and peas; transfer to a small bowl.
4. To the same skillet, add the second ½ teaspoon olive oil. Add chicken and cook about 10 minutes, turning occasionally, until evenly browned.
5. Return vegetables to the skillet; add the ½ cup broth and the thyme; mix lightly.
6. Spoon mixture over bulgur. Cover and bake in preheated oven for 30 minutes.

Estimated nutrients per serving:
Calories: 460
Total protein (grams): 31
Soy protein (grams): 0
Total carbohydrate (grams): 73
Total fat (grams): 6
Total fiber (grams): 17
Total fruit and vegetable (servings): 2, including ½ serving of cruciferous vegetable

For prostate protection: *This recipe cannot be modified to meet the prostate cancer recommendations.*

FAJITAS

Fajitas are traditionally prepared with either chicken or beef and served with sour cream and guacamole. We reduced the fat and added soy protein by using baked tofu. The peppers, onions, and cilantro are familiar flavors in fajitas. In this recipe, they are prepared with a minimum of fat.

YIELD: 2 SERVINGS, 2 FAJITAS EACH
PREPARATION TIME: 15 MINUTES
COOKING TIME: 10 MINUTES

INGREDIENTS:

1 (7-ounce) package baked tofu
¼ cup salsa
1 cup cauliflower florets
1 medium sweet red pepper
1 medium green bell pepper
½ teaspoon olive oil
4 green onions, sliced
4 (8-inch) flour tortillas
1 small tomato, chopped
2 tablespoons cilantro, coarsely chopped

Preheat oven to 350 degrees.

1. Cut tofu into small pieces and combine in a bowl with the salsa; let stand while preparing the vegetables.
2. Cut cauliflower into grape-size pieces and peppers into julienne strips.
3. In a large skillet, heat olive oil over medium heat; add green onions, cauliflower, and peppers. Sauté for 10 minutes, stirring frequently.
4. Add tofu-salsa mixture to the pan; stir gently just to mix.
5. Wrap tortillas in foil and place in the preheated oven for 5 minutes.
6. Remove tortillas from oven. Place mixture in a line along the center of each tortilla; add one-fourth of the chopped tomato and cilantro to each fajita. Fold the bottom of the tortilla over the mixture, fold in the two sides, and fold the remaining side to enclose the mixture.

Estimated nutrients per serving:

Calories: 440
Total protein (grams): 18
Soy protein (grams): 6
Total carbohydrate (grams): 72
Total fat (grams): 9
Total fiber (grams): 9
Total fruit and vegetable (servings): 3, including 1 serving of cruciferous vegetable

For prostate protection: For minimal fat, use ¼ instead of ½ teaspoon olive oil.

MEDITERRANEAN

GREEN CABBAGE STUFFED WITH BULGUR AND VEGETABLES

You may be surprised when you see a whole head of cabbage in the list of ingredients. The best way to remove the leaves intact and undamaged is outlined in the instructions below. The remaining cabbage, even though a little blanched, can be used in many recipes.

YIELD: 2 SERVINGS
PREPARATION TIME: 30 MINUTES
COOKING TIME: 40 MINUTES

INGREDIENTS:
1 head green cabbage
¼ cup bulgur (cracked wheat)
3 tablespoons boiling water
2 tablespoons olive oil
¼ large onion, chopped
2 cloves roasted garlic, minced
3 medium mushrooms, chopped
¼ cup cooked mature soybeans (page 181), or canned soybeans
1 cup diced, cooked butternut squash
1 tablespoon sunflower seeds
2 dried mission figs
¼ teaspoon salt
⅛ teaspoon pepper
⅛ teaspoon powdered cumin
⅛ teaspoon nutmeg
½ cup vegetable stock, homemade (page 88) or canned

Preheat oven to 350 degrees.

1. In a saucepan large enough to hold the head of cabbage, add water until half full. Bring water to a boil. Put the head of cabbage, core side down, into the boiling water. Return to boil and cook for about 3 minutes, until outer leaves are tender.

2. Drain cabbage and cool under cold running water.

3. Carefully, to avoid tearing, peel off four outer leaves. Set aside. Save remaining cabbage for other uses.

4. Place bulgur in a small bowl. Add the 3 tablespoons boiling water and set aside.

5. In a large nonstick skillet, heat olive oil over medium-high heat; add onion and garlic. Cook for 3 minutes, until brown. Add mushrooms; cook for 3 minutes longer. Add soybeans, squash, sunflower seeds, figs, and seasonings. Stir to mix. Add bulgur; stir again to mix.

6. Place one-fourth of the mixture on each of the cabbage leaves. Fold the thick stem over the mixture, fold the sides in and roll. Place seam down in a baking dish. Pour stock over cabbage rolls; cover.

7. Bake in preheated oven for 40 minutes.

Estimated nutrients per serving:

Calories: 440

Total protein (grams): 13

Soy protein (grams): 4

Total carbohydrate (grams): 59

Total fat (grams): 19

Total fiber (grams): 9

Total fruit and vegetable (servings): 3, including 1 serving of cruciferous vegetable

For prostate protection: *For minimal fat, use 1 instead of 2 tablespoons olive oil.*

LINGUINI WITH LENTILS

This unusual combination of lentils and tempeh in a tomato sauce over pasta is unexpectedly delicious and very satisfying. It's great with freshly made pasta.

The lentils, collard greens, and soy tempeh provide a variety of textures and colors.

YIELD: 2 SERVINGS

PREPARATION TIME: 15 MINUTES

COOKING TIME: 25 MINUTES

INGREDIENTS:

4 teaspoons olive oil

½ medium onion, chopped

2 cloves roasted garlic, minced

1 cup tomato sauce

¾ cup vegetable stock, homemade (page 88) or canned

¼ teaspoon oregano

¼ teaspoon basil

¼ teaspoon salt

⅛ teaspoon pepper

½ cup cooked lentils (page 179)

4 ounces soy tempeh, crumbled

3 cups shredded collard greens

4 ounces linguine

2 tablespoons grated Parmesan cheese

1. Heat olive oil over medium heat in a nonstick saucepan.
2. Add onion and garlic and sauté for 5 minutes, until soft.
3. Add tomato sauce, vegetable stock, seasonings, lentils, and tempeh.
4. Bring to boil, reduce heat, and simmer for 10 minutes.
5. In another saucepan, steam the collard greens for 10 minutes; add to sauce. Stir to mix well.
6. Meanwhile, bring 4 quarts of water to a boil. Add ⅛ teaspoon salt and a few drops of olive oil.
7. Add linguini noodles; cook for 15 minutes, until noodles are tender. Drain but do not rinse.
8. Put noodles on plates or into pasta bowls, top with sauce, and sprinkle with Parmesan cheese.

Estimated nutrients per serving:

Calories: 560

Total protein (grams): 27

Soy protein (grams): 11

Total carbohydrate (grams): 81

Total fat (grams): 17

Total fiber (grams): 16

Total fruit and vegetable (servings): 2½, including 1½ servings of cruciferous vegetable

For prostate protection: *For minimal fat, use 2 instead of 4 teaspoons olive oil.*

SWORDFISH KEBOBS

These kebobs are also delicious cooked over hot coals on the barbecue and served over Rice and Kale Pilaf (page 190).

YIELD: 2 SERVINGS
PREPARATION TIME: 30 MINUTES
COOKING TIME: 20 MINUTES

INGREDIENTS:
8 ounces swordfish, ¾ inch thick
2 teaspoons olive oil
2 teaspoons fresh lemon juice
1 large sweet red pepper
2 lemon wedges for garnish

Preheat broiler.

1. Cut swordfish into ¾-inch squares.
2. Combine olive oil and lemon juice in a small bowl; add swordfish and marinate for 10 minutes.
3. Remove stems, seeds, and membranes from pepper; cut into 1-inch squares.
4. Put fish and pepper pieces alternately on 4 skewers; place on a broiler pan.
5. Broil for 10 minutes, turning several times to avoid burning. Place the skewers on plates and garnish with lemon wedges.

Estimated nutrients per serving:
Calories: 190
Total protein (grams): 20
Soy protein (grams): 0
Total carbohydrate (grams): 5
Total fat (grams): 10
Total fiber (grams): 2
Total fruit and vegetable (servings): 1

For prostate protection: *For minimal fat, use 1 instead of 2 teaspoons olive oil.*

LASAGNA

This recipe can be completely assembled and baked up to 2 days ahead of time. Cover and store in the refrigerator. To reheat, bake, covered, for about 1 hour or until bubbling. One of the taste judges described it this way: "This lasagna is FANTASTIC! It's creamy but not heavy. The broccoli adds a wonderful crunch, and the mushrooms and olives a great flavor."

YIELD: 6 SERVINGS

PREPARATION TIME: 1 HOUR

COOKING TIME: 45 MINUTES

INGREDIENTS:

1 tablespoon olive oil

½ large onion, chopped

3 cups sliced mushrooms

2 cloves roasted garlic, minced

3 cups broccoli florets, blanched

¼ cup sliced black olives

1 cup low-fat ricotta cheese

½ cup silken tofu

2 tablespoons packed soy protein powder

¼ teaspoon oregano

¼ teaspoon basil

1 (8-ounce) package whole wheat lasagna noodles

3 cups tomato sauce

12 ounces shredded soy mozzarella

Preheat oven to 350 degrees.

1. Heat olive oil in a nonstick skillet; add onion and cook until soft, about 5 minutes.

2. Add mushrooms and garlic and cook until mushrooms are soft, about 3 minutes longer. Remove from heat and add broccoli and olives. Mix gently.

3. Combine ricotta cheese, tofu, soy protein powder, and herbs in a medium bowl until blended.

4. Bring 4 quarts water and ½ teaspoon olive oil to a boil. Add lasagna noodles and boil 12 minutes or until tender. Drain and rinse under warm water.

5. Moisten the bottom of a 9×9-inch pan with 2 tablespoons of the tomato sauce.

6. Put down a single layer of noodles. Spread with one-third of the ricotta mix, one-third of the vegetables, ⅔ cup tomato sauce, and one-fourth of the mozzarella. Repeat twice.

7. Cover with remaining noodles, tomato sauce, and mozzarella.

8. Bake in a preheated oven for 45 minutes or until bubbling.

Estimated nutrients per serving:
Calories: 330
Total protein (grams): 27
Soy protein (grams): 15
Total carbohydrate (grams): 40
Total fat (grams): 7
Total fiber (grams): 5
Total fruit and vegetable (servings): 3, including 1 serving of cruciferous vegetable

For prostate protection: *For minimal fat, use ½ instead of 1 tablespoon olive oil.*

KUBBUL

This is an adaptation of a traditional Middle Eastern recipe that Barbara often enjoyed in her native Australia.

YIELD: 4 SERVINGS
PREPARATION TIME: 30 MINUTES
COOKING TIME: 30 MINUTES

INGREDIENTS:
1 cup finely ground bulgur (cracked wheat)
¾ cup boiling water
4 teaspoons olive oil
1 medium onion, finely chopped
4 cloves roasted garlic, chopped
4 medium mushrooms, chopped
1 cup chopped canned tomatoes
½ cup juice from canned tomatoes

2 tablespoons raisins
⅛ teaspoon salt
½ teaspoon paprika
1 cup cooked mature soybeans (page 181) or canned soybeans
½ teaspoon salt
⅛ teaspoon pepper
2 teaspoons olive oil
2 tablespoons chopped toasted slivered almonds
½ cup plain nonfat yogurt
¼ cup peeled, finely chopped cucumber

Preheat oven to 350 degrees.

1. Place bulgur in a small bowl. Add boiling water; set aside.
2. Heat the 4 teaspoons olive oil over medium heat in a medium skillet; add onion and cook until golden. Set aside half the onion.
3. To the remaining onion in the skillet, add garlic and mushrooms. Cook until soft.
4. Add tomatoes, juice, raisins, the ⅛ teaspoon salt, and paprika. Set aside.
5. Process the soybeans, reserved onion, ½ teaspoon salt, pepper, and 2 teaspoons olive oil in a food processor until finely chopped. Add soaked bulgur and almonds and process until well blended.
6. Press bulgur mixture firmly into an 8-inch-square baking pan; top with vegetable mixture.
7. Cover and bake in preheated oven for 30 minutes.
8. Combine yogurt and cucumber. Cut kubbul into pieces and serve topped with yogurt-cucumber mixture.

Estimated nutrients per serving:

Calories: 340
Total protein (grams): 16
Soy protein (grams): 7
Total carbohydrate (grams): 45
Total fat (grams): 14
Total fiber (grams): 11
Total fruit and vegetable (servings): 1

For prostate protection: For minimal fat, use 2 instead of 4 teaspoons olive oil in step 2.

BAKED TROUT FILLETS

C apers are small flower buds of a shrub grown in the Mediterranean region. They are usually preserved in vinegar or salt. In this recipe, capers add a complex flavor and contrast well with the fish. This dish hits the spot when you're craving seafood.

YIELD: 2 SERVINGS

PREPARATION TIME: 10 MINUTES

COOKING TIME: 30 MINUTES

INGREDIENTS:
  2 teaspoons olive oil
  ½ cup sliced onion
  ½ cup chopped celery
  ½ cup vegetable stock, homemade (page 88) or canned
  ¼ teaspoon salt
  ⅛ teaspoon pepper
  2 (4-ounce) trout fillets
  ½ tablespoon chopped capers
  1 tablespoon chopped Italian parsley

Preheat oven to 350 degrees.
  1. In a medium nonstick skillet, heat olive oil over medium heat; add onion and celery. Cook for 5 minutes, until onion is golden brown. Add stock; bring to a boil. Add salt and pepper.
  2. Pour mixture into bottom of a flat baking dish large enough to hold the fish without crowding.
  3. Place the fish on top of vegetable mixture. Sprinkle with capers and Italian parsley.
  4. Cover; place in preheated oven. Bake for 20 minutes.
  5. Place fish on 2 individual serving plates. Spoon the vegetables and some of the juice over the fish.

Estimated nutrients per serving:
  Calories: 220
  Total protein (grams): 24
  Soy protein (grams): 0
  Total carbohydrate (grams): 4

Total fat (grams): 12
Total fiber (grams): 1
Total fruit and vegetable (servings): 1

For prostate protection: *For minimal fat, use 1 instead of 2 teaspoons olive oil.*

TRICOLOR PASTA WITH TOMATO AND SOYBEAN SAUCE

Rita used to be teased about cooking with soybeans until she started serving fresh green soybeans to friends. They especially like this quick, easy pasta dish.

YIELD: 2 SERVINGS
PREPARATION TIME: 20 MINUTES
COOKING TIME: 10 MINUTES

INGREDIENTS:

2 teaspoons olive oil
¼ medium onion, chopped
½ medium green bell pepper, stems, seeds, and membranes removed; chopped
4 medium mushrooms, sliced
4 cloves roasted garlic, chopped
½ cup tomato puree
¼ cup vegetable stock, homemade (page 88) or canned
1 cup fresh green soybeans
¼ teaspoon salt
⅛ teaspoon pepper
½ teaspoon dry basil
1 tablespoon chopped Italian parsley
2 cups tricolor spiral pasta
1 tablespoon freshly grated Parmesan cheese

1. In a medium nonstick skillet, heat olive oil over medium heat; add onion. Cook for 5 minutes, until onion is a deep golden brown. Add green pepper, mushrooms, and garlic. Cook for 2 minutes longer, until vegetables are soft.

2. Add tomato puree, stock, soybeans, salt, pepper, and basil. Bring to a boil. Add parsley. Set aside.

3. Meanwhile, bring 4 quarts of water to a boil; add ¼ teaspoon salt and a few drops of olive oil. Add pasta and cook for 8 to 10 minutes, until tender.

4. Drain pasta. Serve topped with sauce and sprinkled with Parmesan cheese.

Estimated nutrients per serving:

Calories: 440

Total protein (grams): 22

Soy protein (grams): 11

Total carbohydrate (grams): 60

Total fat (grams): 13

Total fiber (grams): 8

Total fruit and vegetable (servings): 2

For prostate protection: *For minimal fat, use 1 instead of 2 teaspoons olive oil.*

MAIN-DISH SALADS

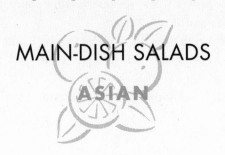

ASIAN

TUNA-ASPARAGUS SALAD

This salad is a visual delight: the delicate, creamy-smooth hearts of palm contrast with the intense colors of the black soybeans and the green asparagus. Hearts of palm, which are the shoots of the palmetto plant, are available canned. Please select dolphin-safe tuna.

YIELD: 2 SERVINGS

PREPARATION TIME: 10 MINUTES

COOKING TIME: 5 MINUTES

INGREDIENTS:

10 medium asparagus spears, tough ends removed, sliced in 1-inch pieces
2 sticks canned hearts of palm, cut into ½-inch slices
1 (6.35-ounce) can prepared black soybeans, rinsed, tangle and
    chestnuts removed
6 ounces canned water-packed albacore tuna or fresh cooked tuna
¼ cup Rice Vinegar Dressing (page 202)
2 cups shredded baby bok choy leaves and stems
2 very thin slices red onion, separated into rings
2 very thin slices lemon

1. Blanch asparagus. Put into large bowl. Add hearts of palm, soybeans, and tuna. Stir gently to combine.
2. Add dressing. Stir gently.
3. Serve on a bed of bok choy and top with onion rings.
4. Garnish with lemon slices.

Estimated nutrients per serving:
Calories: 240
Total protein (grams): 36
Soy protein (grams): 11
Total carbohydrate (grams): 12
Total fat (grams): 7
Total fiber (grams): 6
Total fruit and vegetable (servings): 2, including 1 serving of cruciferous vegetable

For prostate protection: *This recipe cannot be modified to meet the prostate cancer recommendations.*

SPICY NOODLE SALAD

Chinese long beans, sometimes called yard-long beans because they can be up to thirty-six inches long, have a characteristic flavor that goes well in this recipe. Look for them in Asian food markets or grocery stores with a large selection of produce. If you can't find them, substitute ordinary fresh green beans. This is best made ahead to let the flavors blend and develop. Make extra for a workday lunch.

YIELD: 2 SERVINGS
PREPARATION TIME: 20 MINUTES
COOKING TIME: 30 MINUTES

INGREDIENTS:
   6 ounces uncooked thin Chinese egg noodles
   1 tablespoon sesame oil
   1 tablespoon tamari soy sauce
   1 teaspoon rice vinegar
   6 drops chili oil
   1 cup small broccoli florets, blanched
   12 small snow peas, blanched
   ½ cup 1-inch pieces Chinese long beans or other green beans,
      blanched
   1 medium carrot, sliced, blanched
   ½ large sweet red pepper

3½ ounces teriyaki baked tofu
½ teaspoon freshly grated ginger
2 teaspoons chopped cilantro
½ teaspoon sesame seeds, toasted

1. Cook noodles according to package directions. Drain. Place in a large bowl.
2. In a teacup or small bowl, combine sesame oil, soy sauce, vinegar, and chili oil. Pour half of this mixture over noodles. Cover the noodles and set aside.
3. Meanwhile, combine broccoli, snow peas, beans, carrot, red pepper, tofu, and ginger in a medium bowl. Add remaining dressing and toss.
4. Place noodles on 2 individual serving plates; top with vegetable mixture.
5. Sprinkle with cilantro and sesame seeds.
6. Serve at room temperature.

Estimated nutrients per serving:
Calories: 430
Total protein (grams): 17
Soy protein (grams): 4
Total carbohydrate (grams): 67
Total fat (grams): 11
Total fiber (grams): 7
Total fruit and vegetable (servings): 4, including 1 serving of cruciferous vegetable

For prostate protection: *For minimal fat, use ½ instead of 1 tablespoon sesame oil.*

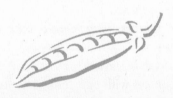

NEW AMERICAN

VEGETABLE-POTATO SALAD

This vegetable-potato salad is a good substitute for the traditional mayonnaise-based potato salad. It is wonderful for potlucks because the vibrant colors add visual appeal to any buffet table. It is equally delicious eaten warm or cold. The salad is a good source of many nutrients, especially folic acid from the asparagus.

YIELD: 2 SERVINGS

PREPARATION TIME: 15 MINUTES

COOKING TIME: 15 MINUTES TO COOK THE POTATOES

INGREDIENTS:

12 (1-inch diameter) red new potatoes
3 tablespoons Balsamic Vinegar Dressing (page 200)
12 stalks asparagus
¼ cup shredded carrot
½ cup shredded red cabbage
¼ medium Fuji apple, sliced
1 tablespoon coarsely chopped curly-leaf parsley
¼ teaspoon salt
12 baby bok choy leaves
½ slice red onion

1. Scrub potatoes (do not peel) and cut into quarters.
2. Cook potatoes in boiling water 15 minutes or until soft. Drain; do not rinse.
3. Put in a large bowl, add dressing while potatoes are hot, and stir gently.
4. Trim tough ends off asparagus; cut into 2-inch pieces on the diagonal. Blanch, then rinse quickly under cold running water to stop cooking. Add to potatoes.
5. Add carrot, red cabbage, apple, parsley, and salt.
6. Line individual plates with baby bok choy leaves; mound half of the warm salad on each plate. Garnish with red onion.

Estimated nutrients per serving:
  Calories: 380
  Total protein (grams): 8
  Soy protein (grams): 0
  Total carbohydrate (grams): 70
  Total fat (grams): 9
  Total fiber (grams): 9
  Total fruit and vegetable (servings): 4, including 1 serving of cruciferous vegetable

For prostate protection: *You can use this recipe as is.*

SPRING ARTICHOKE HEART SALAD

The nutty flavor of the soybeans complements the flavors of the vegetables. The soybeans provide abundant amounts of protein and fiber, and many micronutrients.

YIELD: 2 SERVINGS
PREPARATION TIME: 20 MINUTES
COOKING TIME: NONE

INGREDIENTS:
  1 (14-ounce) can artichoke hearts, cut in halves or quarters
  3 tablespoons Balsamic Vinegar Dressing (page 200)
  1 cup cauliflower florets
  24 small English pea pods
  ¼ large sweet red pepper, sliced crosswise
  4 large mushrooms, sliced
  ½ cup cooked mature soybeans (page 181) or canned soybeans
  1½ cups cooked brown rice (page 178)

1. Combine artichoke hearts and dressing in a medium bowl.
2. Blanch cauliflower and pea pods separately; add to artichoke hearts.
3. Add pepper, mushrooms, and soybeans. Mix gently.
4. Put ¾ cup rice on each of 2 plates. Top each with half of the salad mixture.

Estimated nutrients per serving:
Calories: 420
Total protein (grams): 18
Soy protein (grams): 7
Total carbohydrate (grams): 64
Total fat (grams): 13
Total fiber (grams): 12
Total fruit and vegetable (servings): 5, including 1 serving of cruciferous vegetable

For prostate protection: *You can use this recipe as is.*

SALMON LUNCHEON SALAD

When you grill salmon for dinner (Grilled Salmon with Sesame and Lime, page 150), cook extra to use in this salad. The fat in the salmon has a high percentage of omega-3 fatty acids.

YIELD: 2 SERVINGS
PREPARATION TIME: 10 MINUTES
COOKING TIME: NONE

INGREDIENTS:
2 cups bite-size pieces romaine lettuce
2 cups bite-size pieces red leaf lettuce
¼ cup shredded red cabbage
¼ cup shredded green cabbage
½ cup broccoli florets, blanched
2 tablespoons Lemon Dressing (page 201)
2 medium tomatoes, cut into large chunks
¾ cup fresh green soybeans
6 ounces salmon, cooked or canned, broken into bite-size pieces
1 slice red onion, separated into rings
1 teaspoon capers, chopped

1. Combine lettuces with cabbages and broccoli.
2. Add dressing, toss, and divide between 2 individual plates.
3. Arrange the tomatoes and soybeans on top of salad.
4. Top with salmon; garnish with onion rings and capers.

Estimated nutrients per serving:

Calories: 310

Total protein (grams): 28

Soy protein (grams): 8

Total carbohydrate (grams): 18

Total fat (grams): 15

Total fiber (grams): 7

Total fruit and vegetable (servings): 4, including 1 serving of cruciferous vegetable

For prostate protection: *This recipe cannot be modified to meet the prostate cancer recommendations.*

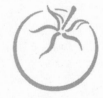

MEDITERRANEAN

SPRING CRACKED WHEAT SALAD

This salad goes together quickly for a delicious lunchtime meal. Cooked or canned soybeans add soy protein to the menu plan.

YIELD: 2 SERVINGS
PREPARATION TIME: 20 MINUTES
COOKING TIME: NONE

INGREDIENTS:
½ cup bulgur (cracked wheat)
6 tablespoons boiling water
8 medium stalks asparagus
1 cup shredded red cabbage
1 medium green onion, chopped
8 walnut halves, quartered
4 small mushrooms
3 tablespoons Balsamic Vinegar Dressing (page 200)
1 cup fresh green soybeans
2 tablespoons crumbled reduced-fat feta cheese

1. Place bulgur in a small bowl. Add the boiling water and set aside.
2. Remove tough ends from asparagus and discard; cut asparagus into long diagonal pieces. Blanch.
3. Combine asparagus, red cabbage, onion, walnuts, mushrooms, and dressing in a bowl. Mix gently.
4. Fluff bulgur with a fork. Stir in soybeans and place on 2 salad plates. Spoon the salad over the bulgur; top with feta cheese.

Estimated nutrients per serving:
Calories: 400
Total protein (grams): 21
Soy protein (grams): 13
Total carbohydrate (grams): 49
Total fat (grams): 16

Total fiber (grams): 14
Total fruit and vegetable (servings): 2, including 1 serving of cruciferous vegetable

For prostate protection: *For minimal dietary fat, use 4 instead of 8 walnut halves.*

ROASTED PEPPERS AND EGGPLANT SALAD

This is one of the first Mediterranean recipes that we developed, and it remains one of our favorites. The rich varied colors of the vegetables makes this a beautiful dish. Eggplant should be salted before cooking to remover excess water and bitterness. Don't be put off by this step. It takes time but not effort.

YIELD: 2 SERVINGS

PREPARATION TIME: 30 MINUTES, PLUS SALTING TIME

COOKING TIME: 40 MINUTES

INGREDIENTS:

1 small eggplant
2 teaspoons salt
2 teaspoons olive oil
1 medium sweet red pepper
1 medium sweet yellow pepper
1 medium green bell pepper
1 small zucchini, sliced, blanched
1 cup cauliflower florets, blanched
2 medium green onions, sliced
¼ cup plain nonfat yogurt
1 tablespoon Lemon Dressing (page 201)
1 teaspoon balsamic vinegar
1 clove roasted garlic, minced
1 tablespoon raisins

Preheat oven to 350 degrees.
  1. Peel the eggplant and cut into ½-inch slices. Spread on a cookie sheet lined with a paper towel. Sprinkle with half of the salt.

When tiny droplets of water form on the surface of the eggplant, turn the eggplant slices over and sprinkle with remaining salt. Let stand 1 hour, then rinse eggplant slices and pat dry.

2. Place the eggplant slices on a cookie sheet. Brush both sides of the eggplant with the 2 teaspoons olive oil. Bake for 40 minutes, turning over after 20 minutes.

3. Cut the peppers in half lengthwise; remove stems, seeds, and membranes. Place cut side down on a cookie sheet. Bake for 30 minutes. Remove peppers from oven and cool enough to handle.

4. Remove any loose skin from peppers, cut in half lengthwise again, and cut into ½-inch slices.

5. Cut the eggplant into chunks.

6. Place all vegetables in a bowl; mix gently.

7. In a small bowl, combine yogurt, dressing, vinegar, and garlic. Mix well. Add to vegetables and mix gently.

8. Serve topped with raisins.

Estimated nutrients per serving:

Calories: 230
Total protein (grams): 7
Soy protein (grams): 0
Total carbohydrate (grams): 37
Total fat (grams): 8
Total fiber (grams): 10
Total fruit and vegetable (servings): 7, including 1 serving of cruciferous vegetable

For prostate protection: *You can use this recipe as is.*

ANTIPASTO

A Mediterranean section of a cookbook wouldn't be complete without antipasto. We developed this recipe to be served as an entrée instead of before a pasta course, as its name suggests.

YIELD: 2 SERVINGS
PREPARATION TIME: 15 MINUTES
COOKING TIME: NONE

INGREDIENTS:
½ medium sweet yellow pepper, stems, seeds, and membranes removed
½ medium green bell pepper, stems, seeds, and membranes removed
1 large Roma tomato, sliced lengthwise
8 large Kalamata olives
2 ounces low-fat mozzarella cheese, sliced
1 cup Marinated Cauliflower (page 217), well drained
4 sticks hearts of palm
¼ cup Soybean Hummus (page 182)

1. Arrange all ingredients except hummus on a serving platter.
2. Serve hummus in a small bowl and use as a dip for the vegetables or a spread for French bread.

Estimated nutrients per serving:
Calories: 230
Total protein (grams): 15
Soy protein (grams): 4
Total carbohydrate (grams): 16
Total fat (grams): 13
Total fiber (grams): 6
Total fruit and vegetable (servings): 2

For prostate protection: *For minimal dietary fat, use 4 instead of 8 olives.*

VEGETABLE AND BARLEY SALAD

This hearty salad makes a welcome addition to potluck meals because it provides an alternative for people choosing to increase whole grains and fruits and vegetables and limit meat consumption. Quantities can easily be doubled or tripled.

YIELD: 2 SERVINGS
PREPARATION TIME: 15 MINUTES
COOKING TIME: NONE

INGREDIENTS:
½ medium sweet red pepper
1 cup cooked barley (page 180)

1 cup thinly sliced baby bok choy stems
¼ cup green peas
2 medium green onions, sliced
½ cup canned soybeans or cooked mature soybeans (page 181)
2 tablespoons slivered almonds, toasted
2 large fresh basil leaves, chopped
3 tablespoons Lemon Dressing (page 201)

1. Remove stems, seeds, and membranes from pepper; rinse. Slice into thin strips.
2. Combine all ingredients except dressing in a large bowl.
3. Add dressing and mix gently.

Estimated nutrients per serving:
Calories: 320
Total protein (grams): 12
Soy protein (grams): 7
Total carbohydrate (grams): 33
Total fat (grams): 15
Total fiber (grams): 10
Total fruit and vegetable (servings): 2, including 1 serving of cruciferous vegetable

For prostate protection: For minimal dietary fat, use 1 instead of 2 tablespoons almonds.

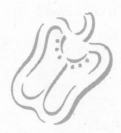

SIDE DISHES — GRAINS AND LEGUMES
BASIC RECIPES

COOKED BROWN RICE

Cooked brown rice is a "staple" in many of the recipes in this book. You can make it ahead in quantity and keep it in the refrigerator for several days to have on hand.

YIELD: ABOUT 3 CUPS
PREPARATION TIME: 5 MINUTES
COOKING TIME: 50 MINUTES

INGREDIENTS:
2¼ cups water
1 cup long-grain brown rice

1. In a medium saucepan, bring water to a boil.
2. Add rice; stir. Reduce heat, cover, and cook for 50 minutes or until water is absorbed. Do not stir while rice is cooking.

Estimated nutrients per cup:
Calories: 220
Total protein (grams): 5
Soy protein (grams): 0
Total carbohydrate (grams): 45
Total fat (grams): 2
Total fiber (grams): 4

For prostate protection: *You can use this recipe as is.*

COOKED WILD RICE

Wild rice, also known as water oats, comes from the rich tradition of Native Americans. It is not actually rice; it's a wild grass seed, which continues to be grown along the edges of lakes in the northern United States and harvested by Native Americans. Its intriguing, nutty flavor and unique texture are a great addition to many dishes.

YIELD: ABOUT 3 CUPS
PREPARATION TIME: 5 MINUTES
COOKING TIME: 40 TO 50 MINUTES

INGREDIENTS:
  3 cups water
  1 cup wild rice

1. In a medium saucepan, bring water to a boil.
2. Add wild rice, stir. Reduce heat, cover, and cook for 40 to 50 minutes or until water is absorbed. Do not stir while rice is cooking.

Estimated nutrients per cup:
  Calories: 160
  Total protein (grams): 7
  Soy protein (grams): 0
  Total carbohydrate (grams): 35
  Total fat (grams): 1
  Total fiber (grams): 3

For prostate protection: *You can use this recipe as is.*

COOKED LENTILS

This high-protein food is rich in many B vitamins, minerals, and fiber. It is good mixed with rice and in soups and stews.

YIELD: ABOUT 2½ CUPS
PREPARATION TIME: 5 MINUTES
COOKING TIME: 20 MINUTES

INGREDIENTS:
1 cup dry lentils
6 cups water

1. Wash lentils under cold running water and discard any debris.
2. Combine lentils and water in a large saucepan. Bring to a boil.
3. Reduce heat, cover, and cook for 35 to 45 minutes or until tender but not mushy.
4. Drain and use in recipes as directed.

Estimated nutrients per ½ cup:
Calories: 110
Total protein (grams): 9
Soy protein (grams): 0
Total carbohydrate (grams): 20
Total fat (grams): 0
Total fiber (grams): 8

For prostate protection: *You can use this recipe as is.*

· COOKED BARLEY

Although barley is most commonly used for making beer, it is delicious as a cooked grain. It is also great in soups, stews, and other mixed dishes. It is available as either pearl barley (polished) or Scotch barley (husked and ground).

YIELD: ABOUT 1¾ CUPS
PREPARATION TIME: 5 MINUTES
COOKING TIME: 45 MINUTES

INGREDIENTS:
½ cup pearl barley
3 cups water

1. Rinse barley under running water.
2. In a medium saucepan, bring the 3 cups water to a boil.

3. Add barley, stir, and bring water back to a boil. Reduce heat, cover, and cook for 45 minutes or until water is absorbed. Do not stir during cooking.

Estimated nutrients per ½ cup:
Calories: 100
Total protein (grams): 2
Soy protein (grams): 0
Total carbohydrate (grams): 22
Total fat (grams): 0
Total fiber (grams): 4

For prostate protection: *You can use this recipe as is.*

COOKED MATURE SOYBEANS OR OTHER BEANS

Different types of beans have been a staple of the diets of many cultures for centuries. There are many types of beans available. The common varieties are readily available canned or dried in large grocery stores. Look for the more unusual varieties (like the Christmas beans in the Three-Bean Chili) in specialty stores and where grains and legumes are sold in bulk. Beans have long been recognized for their protein, fiber, iron, and B vitamins.

This method of cooking beans eliminates the need to soak them overnight. The instructions here can be used for all varieties of beans. Discarding the initial soaking liquid will get rid of most of the compounds that cause gastrointestinal gas in many people.

YIELD: ABOUT 4 CUPS
PREPARATION TIME: 5 MINUTES
COOKING TIME: VARIES

INGREDIENTS:
1 cup dried mature soybeans or other beans
Water as needed

1. Rinse beans well and discard any debris.
2. Put beans in a heavy saucepan; cover with plenty of water (to 2

inches above the beans). Bring to a boil, cover, remove from heat, and let stand for 1 hour.

3. Drain soaking liquid and rinse beans with cold water.
4. Return to pan; cover with fresh water to 2 inches above the beans. Bring to a boil, cover, reduce heat, and cook for 30 minutes to 2 hours or until tender. If all the water is absorbed before the beans are cooked, add boiling water as needed. (Cooking time depends on the type of bean.)

Use in recipes as directed.

Estimated nutrients per ½ cup soybeans:
Calories: 150
Total protein (grams): 14
Soy protein (grams): 14
Total carbohydrate (grams): 9
Total fat (grams): 8
Total fiber (grams): 5

For prostate protection: *You can use this recipe as is.*

SOYBEAN HUMMUS

This recipe uses soybeans instead of chickpeas as a base. We feature it in several of the recipes. It's great as an appetizer on pita bread wedges or as a "dip" for a variety of fresh vegetables. If you want to spice it up, consider adding fresh ground garlic or a little more lemon juice.

YIELD: 1 CUP
PREPARATION TIME: 5 MINUTES
COOKING TIME: NONE

INGREDIENTS:
1 cup cooked mature soybeans (page 181) or canned soybeans
1 teaspoon tahini
5 teaspoons lemon juice
1 tablespoon olive oil
4 drops sesame oil

2 tablespoons water
⅛ teaspoon cayenne

1. Put all ingredients in a blender.
2. Process until smooth.
3. Use in recipes as directed or enjoy as a dip for vegetables or a spread for pita bread or flatbread.

Estimated nutrients per 2 tablespoons:
    Calories: 60
    Total protein (grams): 4
    Soy protein (grams): 4
    Total carbohydrate (grams): 2
    Total fat (grams): 4
    Total fiber (grams): 1
    Total fruit and vegetable (servings): none

For prostate protection: *You can use this recipe as is.*

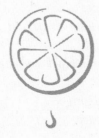

ASIAN

FRIED RICE WITH SHRIMP

Fried rice has always been a well-known and popular Chinese rice dish. There are many versions. Ours uses prepared black soybeans, which provide fabulous flavor and visual appeal. One of the judges commented: "This really tastes grrrrrreat! I love it and would have it as a main course as well as a side dish."

YIELD: 2 SERVINGS

PREPARATION TIME: 15 MINUTES

COOKING TIME: 15 MINUTES

INGREDIENTS:

1 tablespoon canola oil
1 medium green onion, chopped
2 cloves roasted garlic, minced
¼ medium green bell pepper, sliced
¼ medium sweet red pepper, sliced
1 cup cooked brown rice (page 178), cold
1 cup cooked white rice, cold
1 (6.35-ounce) can prepared black soybeans, rinsed, tangle and
　chestnuts removed
⅛ teaspoon freshly grated ginger
⅛ teaspoon tamari soy sauce
8 drops chili oil
½ cup cooked baby shrimp
1 (1-inch) piece green onion, thinly sliced lengthwise

1. In a medium skillet or wok, heat canola oil over medium-high heat. Add green onion, garlic, green and red peppers. Cook for 2 minutes, stirring constantly.
2. Add brown and white rice. Cook for 4 minutes, stirring constantly.
3. Add soybeans, ginger, soy sauce, and chili oil. Cook for 2 minutes longer, stirring constantly and gently.

4. Add shrimp and cook until heated thoroughly.
5. Serve topped with green onion.

Estimated nutrients per serving:
Calories: 430
Total protein (grams): 22
Soy protein (grams): 11
Total carbohydrate (grams): 54
Total fat (grams): 14
Total fiber (grams): 7
Total fruit and vegetable (servings): 1

For prostate protection:
▪ *To eliminate animal products, omit shrimp.*
▪ *For minimal dietary fat, use ½ instead of 1 tablespoon canola oil.*

NEW AMERICAN

CORN BREAD

Corn bread is a staple in many households and each household has a favorite recipe. We use corn kernels to provide a textural contrast. The nutty flavor of soy flour lends itself to this bread. Soy flour is a good source of soy protein.

YIELD: 6 SERVINGS
PREPARATION TIME: 30 MINUTES
COOKING TIME: 30 MINUTES

INGREDIENTS:
½ cup soy flour
½ cup whole wheat flour
1 tablespoon baking powder
½ teaspoon salt
1 cup cornmeal
½ cup brown sugar
1 large egg
4 tablespoons light olive oil
1 cup nonfat soy milk
½ cup frozen corn

Preheat oven to 350 degrees.
1. Sift together soy flour, whole wheat flour, baking powder, and salt. Stir in cornmeal and brown sugar.
2. In a small bowl, lightly beat the egg with a fork. Beat in the olive oil; stir in the soy milk.
3. Add corn; mix lightly to combine.
4. Make a well in the dry ingredients. Pour liquid mixture into well. Stir until just mixed.
5. Pour into nonstick 8×8-inch pan.
6. Bake in preheated oven for 30 minutes.
7. Cool in pan on a cooling rack for 5 to 10 minutes before removing from pan.

Estimated nutrients per serving:

Calories: 340

Total protein (grams): 10

Soy protein (grams): 4

Total carbohydrate (grams): 53

Total fat (grams): 11

Total fiber (grams): 5

Total fruit and vegetable (servings): none

For prostate protection: *This recipe cannot be modified to meet the prostate cancer recommendations.*

QUINOA

This grain (pronounced *keen-wa*) from the Andes is grown only at elevations between seven thousand and eleven thousand feet. Its caviar-like texture has earned it the sobriquet "caviar of grains." Quinoa is a good source of high-quality protein and has a delicate taste. Enjoy it as an alternative to rice or pasta. It has a crunchy texture and is especially good with fish.

YIELD: 2 SERVINGS

PREPARATION TIME: 5 MINUTES

COOKING TIME: 15 MINUTES

INGREDIENTS:

½ cup quinoa

1 cup water

1. Put quinoa in a bowl and rinse thoroughly with cold water several times. Drain and put into a small saucepan with 1 cup water.
2. Bring to a boil. Cover, reduce heat, and simmer for about 15 minutes, until grains are transparent and all water is absorbed.
3. Remove from heat and fluff with a fork.

Estimated nutrients per serving:

Calories: 320

Total protein (grams): 11

Soy protein (grams): 0
Total carbohydrate (grams): 59
Total fat (grams): 5
Total fiber (grams): 5
Total fruit and vegetable (servings): none

For prostate protection: *You can use this recipe as is.*

MIXED-GRAIN PILAF

This pilaf is easy and goes together quickly. Because the recipe uses whole grains, it takes a long time to cook. The flavor of the whole grains is worth waiting for. While the pilaf is cooking, prepare the remainder of the dinner.

YIELD: 2 SERVINGS
PREPARATION TIME: 15 MINUTES
COOKING TIME: 50 MINUTES

INGREDIENTS:
  1 teaspoon olive oil
  ½ medium onion, chopped
  2 cloves roasted garlic, crushed
  ¼ cup uncooked brown rice
  ¼ cup uncooked pearl barley
  1¼ cups vegetable stock, homemade (page 88) or canned
  3 tablespoons boiling water
  ¼ cup uncooked bulgur

1. In a saucepan, heat the olive oil over medium heat. Add onion and garlic and cook for 5 minutes. Add rice and barley and continue to cook 5 minutes longer.
2. Add vegetable broth. Bring to a boil, reduce heat, cover, and cook for 40 minutes.
3. Meanwhile, pour the boiling water over the bulgur in a small bowl. Set aside.
4. When rice mixture has cooked for 40 minutes, stir in bulgur. Cook for 10 minutes longer.
5. Fluff with a fork and serve.

Estimated nutrients per serving:

    Calories: 280

    Total protein (grams): 7

    Soy protein (grams): 0

    Total carbohydrate (grams): 56

    Total fat (grams): 3.5

    Total fiber (grams): 9

    Total fruit and vegetable (servings): none

For prostate protection: *For minimal dietary fat, use ½ instead of 1 teaspoon olive oil.*

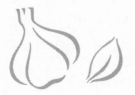

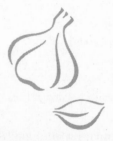

MEDITERRANEAN

RICE AND KALE PILAF

Plan ahead to have some cooked brown rice available for this dish. Kale, a cruciferous vegetable, lends color and flavor to the brown rice.

YIELD: 2 SERVINGS
PREPARATION TIME: 10 MINUTES
COOKING TIME: 12 MINUTES

INGREDIENTS:
> 2 cups finely shredded kale leaves
> 1½ cups cooked brown rice (page 178)
> 1 tablespoon toasted pine nuts
> Pinch nutmeg
> Pinch salt
> 2 teaspoons olive oil

1. Steam kale for 10 minutes.
2. Add cooked brown rice, pine nuts, nutmeg, salt, and olive oil. Fluff with a fork.
3. Heat gently for about 3 minutes or until hot.

Estimated nutrients per serving:
Calories: 250
Total protein (grams): 6
Soy protein (grams): 0
Total carbohydrate (grams): 38
Total fat (grams): 9
Total fiber (grams): 5
Total fruit and vegetable (servings): 1, including 1 serving of cruciferous vegetable

For prostate protection: *For minimal dietary fat, use 1 instead of 2 teaspoons olive oil.*

SAUTÉED SOYBEANS

For this recipe, be sure to cook the onion to a deep golden brown to bring out its sweetness.

YIELD: 2 SERVINGS
PREPARATION TIME: 5 MINUTES
COOKING TIME: 10 MINUTES

INGREDIENTS:
  1 teaspoon olive oil
  ¼ medium onion, chopped
  ¼ cup sweet red pepper strips
  2 cloves roasted garlic, chopped
  1 cup cooked mature soybeans (page 181) or canned soybeans
  2 tablespoons sliced olives
  4 leaves fresh basil, chopped
  ⅛ teaspoon salt
  Pinch pepper

1. In a medium nonstick skillet, heat olive oil over medium-high heat. Add onion; cook for 5 minutes or until onion is a deep golden brown. Add red pepper and garlic; cook for 2 minutes longer.
2. Add soybeans, olives, basil, salt, and pepper. Stir gently over heat for 2 to 3 minutes.

Estimated nutrients per serving:
  Calories: 190
  Total protein (grams): 15
  Soy protein (grams): 14
  Total carbohydrate (grams): 11
  Total fat (grams): 11
  Total fiber (grams): 6
  Total fruit and vegetable (servings): none

For prostate protection: *For minimal dietary fat, use ½ instead of 1 teaspoon olive oil; use 1 instead of 2 tablespoons sliced olives.*

SIDE DISHES — VEGETABLES
BASIC RECIPE

STEAMED COLLARD GREENS OR KALE

Green leafy vegetables that are usually considered tough become tender when finely shredded and cooked according to this recipe. You can use this method for other greens, like turnip greens or mustard greens, but cooking time may be different. The addition of a tiny amount of olive oil sweetens the greens. Spinach and Swiss chard are tender greens and cook quickly without being shredded.

YIELD: 1 CUP
PREPARATION TIME: 10 MINUTES
COOKING TIME: 10 MINUTES

INGREDIENTS:
  2 cups finely shredded collard greens or kale
  2 tablespoons water
  ¼ teaspoon olive oil

To cook in a saucepan:
  1. Place the greens and water in a heavy saucepan.
  2. Bring to a boil. Reduce heat, cover, and cook for 10 minutes.
  3. Drain. Mix in olive oil.

To cook in a steamer:
  1. Place the greens in top of a steamer.
  2. Steam for 10 minutes.
  3. Mix in olive oil.

Estimated nutrients per serving:

    Calories: 30
    Total protein (grams): 2
    Soy protein (grams): 0
    Total carbohydrate (grams): 4
    Total fat (grams): 1
    Total fiber (grams): 1
    Total fruit and vegetable (servings): 1, including 1 cruciferous vegetable

For prostate protection: *You can use this recipe as is.*

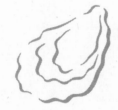

ASIAN

FRESH VEGETABLE MEDLEY

We chose the vegetables for this stir-fry recipe to complement the flavor of the Grilled Fresh Tuna, page 134.

YIELD: 2 SERVINGS
PREPARATION TIME: 15 MINUTES
COOKING TIME: 15 MINUTES

INGREDIENTS:

½ tablespoon cornstarch
¼ cup cold water
4 drops chili oil
1 teaspoon canola oil
¼ cup chopped onion
½ cup small broccoli florets
½ cup small cauliflower florets
½ cup diagonally sliced snow peas
¾ cup fresh green soybeans
¼ medium sweet red pepper, cut in ½-inch pieces
¼ cup sliced water chestnuts
2 cups cooked brown rice (page 178)

1. In a small bowl, mix cornstarch with the water to a smooth paste. Add chili oil. Stir and set aside.
2. In a medium skillet or wok, heat canola oil over medium-high heat. Add onion and cook for 3 minutes.
3. Add broccoli, cauliflower, snow peas, and soybeans. Cook for 3 minutes longer.
4. Add red pepper and water chestnuts. Cook for 2 minutes.
5. Pour cornstarch mixture over the vegetables. Bring to a boil, stirring constantly.
6. Serve over brown rice.

Estimated nutrients per serving:
Calories: 380
Total protein (grams): 16
Soy protein (grams): 8
Total carbohydrate (grams): 65
Total fat (grams): 9
Total fiber (grams): 9
Total fruit and vegetable (servings): 2, including 1 serving of cruciferous vegetable

For prostate protection:
▪ *To increase lycopene, add 8 medium cherry tomatoes at the end of step 5.*
▪ *For minimal dietary fat, use ½ instead of 1 teaspoon canola oil.*

WILTED BABY BOK CHOY

This recipe was created to combine the sweetness of the button mushrooms and the delicate bitterness of the baby bok choy. It lends itself to the small, baby bok choy instead of the regular bok choy. For best results, have the ingredients ready and cook just before serving.

YIELD: 2 SERVINGS
PREPARATION TIME: 10 MINUTES
COOKING TIME: 5 MINUTES

INGREDIENTS:
1 teaspoon canola oil
3 cups chopped baby bok choy
6 small button mushrooms, sliced
2 teaspoons sunflower seeds, toasted
¼ teaspoon white vinegar
½ teaspoon tamari soy sauce
6 drops chili oil

1. In a small skillet or wok, heat canola oil over medium-high heat. Add bok choy, mushrooms, and sunflower seeds. Cook for about 3 minutes or until bok choy is wilted, stirring constantly.
2. Add vinegar, soy sauce, and chili oil. Stir to combine.

Estimated nutrients per serving:
  Calories: 60
  Total protein (grams): 3
  Soy protein (grams): 0
  Total carbohydrate (grams): 4
  Total fat (grams): 4
  Total fiber (grams): 2
  Total fruit and vegetable (servings): 2, including 1½ servings of cruciferous
    vegetable

For prostate protection: *For minimal dietary fat, use ½ instead of 1 tea-spoon canola oil; omit sunflower seeds.*

STEAMED CAULIFLOWER AND FRESH SOYBEANS

This is a cruciferous-soy version of "mixed vegetables."

YIELD: 2 SERVINGS
PREPARATION TIME: 10 MINUTES
COOKING TIME: 5 MINUTES

INGREDIENTS:
  1 cup small cauliflower florets
  ½ cup diced carrot
  ¾ cup fresh green soybeans

1. Steam cauliflower and carrot for 5 minutes.
2. Add soybeans and steam for 5 minutes longer.

Estimated nutrients per serving:
  Calories: 110
  Total protein (grams): 10
  Soy protein (grams): 8
  Total carbohydrate (grams): 13
  Total fat (grams): 5
  Total fiber (grams): 5
  Total fruit and vegetable (servings): 1½, including 1 serving of cruciferous
    vegetable

For prostate protection: *You can use this recipe as is.*

NEW AMERICAN

LEMON CARROTS AND COLLARD GREENS

In this recipe the greens are sweetened by the addition of a tiny amount of olive oil. Make sure the collard greens are finely shredded so they become tender when they are cooked. If the collards taste bitter, you'll find they improve with more olive oil.

YIELD: 2 SERVINGS

PREPARATION TIME: 10 MINUTES

COOKING TIME: 15 MINUTES

INGREDIENTS:

2 cups finely shredded collard greens
1 medium carrot, thinly sliced
¼ teaspoon olive oil
1 teaspoon fresh lemon juice
Pinch dill weed

1. Put the collard greens in a saucepan; steam for 5 minutes.
2. Add carrot; steam for 5 minutes longer.
3. Add olive oil, lemon juice, and dill. Stir gently.

Estimated nutrients per serving:

Calories: 30
Total protein (grams): 1
Soy protein (grams): 0
Total carbohydrate (grams): 6
Total fat (grams): 0
Total fiber (grams): 2
Total fruit and vegetable (servings): 1½, including 1 serving cruciferous vegetables

For prostate protection: *You can use this recipe as is.*

MEDITERRANEAN

BAKED ROMA TOMATOES WITH FRESH BASIL

One of the judges was especially impressed with this simple yet elegant presentation. She said: "It's spectacular. One bite of this tomato-basil combination takes you straight to Italy. The warmth of the tomato is very soothing and the touch of olive oil satisfying. It's a perfect accompaniment to any dish."

YIELD: 2 SERVINGS
PREPARATION TIME: 5 MINUTES
COOKING TIME: 15 MINUTES

INGREDIENTS:
  2 medium Roma tomatoes
  1 teaspoon extra-virgin olive oil
  Pinch salt
  Sprinkle pepper
  1 tablespoon chopped fresh basil

Preheat oven to 350 degrees.
  1. Cut tomatoes in half lengthwise. Place cut side up on baking pan.
  2. Drizzle with olive oil; sprinkle with salt and pepper.
  3. Bake in preheated oven for 10 to 15 minutes.
  4. Remove from oven, sprinkle with basil.

Estimated nutrients per serving:
  Calories: 40
  Total protein (grams): 0
  Soy protein (grams): 0
  Total carbohydrate (grams): 2
  Total fat (grams): 3
  Total fiber (grams): 0
  Total fruit and vegetable (servings): 1

For prostate protection: *For minimal dietary fat, use ½ instead of 1 teaspoon olive oil.*

SICILIAN CABBAGE

This gets rave reviews every time we serve it. When you're going to serve it to company, make sure you have plenty. This is best served as soon as the cabbage is wilted. You can have the ingredients ready ahead of time and cook it at the last minute.

YIELD: 2 SERVINGS

PREPARATION TIME: 10 MINUTES

COOKING TIME: 5 TO 10 MINUTES

INGREDIENTS:

1 teaspoon olive oil
1 tablespoon pine nuts
1 cup shredded cabbage
1 tablespoon sliced olives
1 tablespoon currants

1. In a small saucepan, heat the oil over medium heat. Add pine nuts; cook until golden, stirring constantly to avoid burning.
2. Add cabbage; stir until it is well coated with oil. Add olives and currants; cover and cook for 3 to 5 minutes, until cabbage is just wilted but still crisp. Do not overcook. Serve immediately.

Estimated nutrients per serving:

Calories: 75
Total protein (grams): 1
Soy protein (grams): 0
Total carbohydrate (grams): 7
Total fat (grams): 5
Total fiber (grams): 2
Total fruit and vegetable (servings): 1, including 1 serving of cruciferous vegetable

For prostate protection: *For minimal dietary fat, use ½ instead of 1 teaspoon olive oil; use ½ instead of 1 tablespoon pine nuts.*

SIDE SALADS

SALAD DRESSING BASIC RECIPES

BALSAMIC VINEGAR DRESSING

YIELD: 1¼ CUPS
PREPARATION TIME: 3 MINUTES
COOKING TIME: NONE

INGREDIENTS:
½ cup extra-virgin olive oil
¼ cup balsamic vinegar
½ cup apple juice

1. Place all ingredients in a small jar. Shake well to combine; toss with salad greens or use in recipes as directed.
2. If making in advance, refrigerate and bring to room temperature before using.

Estimated nutrients per tablespoon:
Calories: 50
Total protein (grams): 0
Soy protein (grams): 0
Total carbohydrate (grams): 1
Total fat (grams): 5
Total fiber (grams): 0

For prostate protection: *You can use this recipe as is.*

LEMON DRESSING

YIELD: 1¼ CUPS
PREPARATION TIME: 5 MINUTES
COOKING TIME: NONE

INGREDIENTS:
  ½ cup extra-virgin olive oil
  ¼ cup fresh lemon juice
  ½ cup apple juice

1. Place all ingredients in a small jar. Shake well to combine; toss with salad greens or use in recipes as directed.
2. If making in advance, refrigerate and bring to room temperature before using.

Estimated nutrients per tablespoon:
  Calories: 50
  Total protein (grams): 0
  Soy protein (grams): 0
  Total carbohydrate (grams): 1
  Total fat (grams): 5
  Total fiber (grams): 0

For prostate protection: *You can use this recipe as is.*

TANGY TOFU DRESSING

YIELD: 1 CUP
PREPARATION TIME: 5 MINUTES
COOKING TIME: NONE

INGREDIENTS:
  1 cup silken tofu
  1 tablespoon extra-virgin olive oil
  2 tablespoons cider vinegar

1. Blend silken tofu and olive oil in a blender or food processor until smooth.

2. Add vinegar and blend until all ingredients are well mixed.
3. Use in recipes as directed.
4. If making ahead, refrigerate until needed.

Estimated nutrients per tablespoon:
Calories: 15
Total protein (grams): 1
Soy protein (grams): 0
Total carbohydrate (grams): 0
Total fat (grams): 1
Total fiber (grams): 0

For prostate protection: *You can use this recipe as is.*

RICE VINEGAR DRESSING

YIELD: 1¼ CUPS
PREPARATION TIME: 5 MINUTES
COOKING TIME: NONE

INGREDIENTS:
½ *cup canola oil*
¼ *cup seasoned rice-wine vinegar*
½ *cup apple juice*

1. Place all ingredients in a small jar; shake well to combine. Toss with salad greens or use in recipes as directed.
2. If making in advance, refrigerate and bring to room temperature before using.

Estimated nutrients per tablespoon:
Calories: 50
Total protein (grams): 0
Soy protein (grams): 0
Total carbohydrate (grams): 1
Total fat (grams): 5
Total fiber (grams): 0

For prostate protection: *You can use this recipe as is.*

ASIAN

CARROT-DAIKON SALAD

Daikon is Japanese white radish used extensively in a variety of dishes. Carrot-Daikon Salad is a traditional Japanese dish.

YIELD: 2 SERVINGS
PREPARATION TIME: 10 MINUTES, PLUS 1 HOUR OF CHILLING TIME
COOKING TIME: NONE

INGREDIENTS:
   1 cup grated carrots
   ½ cup grated peeled daikon
   ¼ teaspoon freshly grated ginger
   1 tablespoon rice vinegar
   ¼ teaspoon fish sauce
   1 tablespoon orange juice

1. In a medium bowl, combine carrots, daikon, and ginger.
2. In a small bowl or teacup, make dressing by combining vinegar, fish sauce, and orange juice.
3. Add dressing to vegetables. Stir to combine. Cover and refrigerate for about 1 hour to blend flavors.

Estimated nutrients per serving:
   Calories: 30
   Total protein (grams): 1
   Soy protein (grams): 0
   Total carbohydrate (grams): 7
   Total fat (grams): 0
   Total fiber (grams): 2
   Total fruit and vegetable (servings): 1½

For prostate protection: *You can use this recipe as is.*

WATERCRESS SALAD

YIELD: 2 SERVINGS
PREPARATION TIME: 15 MINUTES, PLUS 1 HOUR OF
CHILLING TIME
COOKING TIME: NONE

INGREDIENTS:
2 cups watercress leaves
½ cup peeled, diced cucumber
¼ cup grated carrot
1 tablespoon rice vinegar
¼ teaspoon tamari soy sauce
1 tablespoon slivered almonds, toasted

1. Blanch the watercress. Squeeze out the liquid.
2. In a medium bowl, combine watercress, cucumber, and carrot.
3. Gently stir in vinegar and soy sauce.
4. Cover and refrigerate for about 1 hour.
5. Serve sprinkled with almonds.

Estimated nutrients per serving:
Calories: 40
Total protein (grams): 2
Soy protein (grams): 0
Total carbohydrate (grams): 4
Total fat (grams): 2
Total fiber (grams): 2
Total fruit and vegetable (servings): 1½, including 1 serving of cruciferous
vegetable

For prostate protection: *For minimal dietary fat, omit almonds.*

ASPARAGUS AND RADISH SALAD

YIELD: 2 SERVINGS
PREPARATION TIME: 10 MINUTES, PLUS 20
MINUTES TO MARINATE
COOKING TIME: NONE

INGREDIENTS:

8 *spears asparagus, tough ends removed, cut in 1½-inch diagonal pieces*
1 *cup small cauliflower florets*
2 *small red radishes, thinly sliced*
2 *tablespoons Rice Vinegar Dressing (page 202)*
½ *teaspoon toasted sesame seeds*

1. Blanch asparagus and cauliflower separately. Place vegetables in a small bowl with radishes.
2. Pour dressing over vegetables while they are still warm; stir gently.
3. Let sit for at least 20 minutes, stirring occasionally.
4. Serve at room temperature, or refrigerate and serve chilled.
5. Top with sesame seeds just before serving.

Estimated nutrients per serving:

Calories 60
Total protein (grams): 3
Soy protein (grams): 0
Total carbohydrate (grams): 6
Total fat (grams): 3
Total fiber (grams): 2
Total fruit and vegetable (servings): 1½, including 1 serving of cruciferous vegetable

For prostate protection: *For minimal dietary fat, omit sesame seeds.*

BEAN SPROUT SALAD

YIELD: 2 SERVINGS
PREPARATION TIME: 10 MINUTES, PLUS 1 HOUR OF CHILLING TIME
COOKING TIME: NONE

INGREDIENTS:

1 *cup mung bean sprouts, coarsely chopped*
9 *medium snow peas, strings removed, thinly sliced on the diagonal, blanched*
2 *tablespoons sliced green onion, green part only*

3 tablespoons rice vinegar
1 teaspoon tamari soy sauce
½ teaspoon sesame oil
1 sprig cilantro, coarsely chopped

1. Rinse bean sprouts in a colander, then pour boiling water over them. Rinse again under cold water. Drain; place in a medium bowl.
2. Add blanched snow peas, green onion, vinegar, soy sauce, and sesame oil. Stir gently to combine.
3. Cover and refrigerate for about 1 hour.
4. Serve sprinkled with cilantro.

Estimated nutrients per serving:
Calories: 30
Total protein (grams): 1.5
Soy protein (grams): 0
Total carbohydrate (grams): 3.5
Total fat (grams): 1
Total fiber (grams): 1
Total fruit and vegetable (servings): 1½

For prostate protection: You can use this recipe as is.

CELERY AND WATER CHESTNUT SALAD

Blanching brings out the bright green color in the celery and the crispness in the water chestnuts.

YIELD: 2 SERVINGS
PREPARATION TIME: 10 MINUTES, PLUS 1 HOUR OF CHILLING TIME
COOKING TIME: NONE

INGREDIENTS:
4 large celery stalks
½ cup water chestnuts
1 teaspoon tamari soy sauce
½ teaspoon sesame oil

1. Trim the celery stalks and slice them thinly on the diagonal. Blanch.
2. Blanch the water chestnuts. Chop coarsely.
3. In a medium bowl, combine celery and water chestnuts.
4. Add soy sauce and sesame oil. Stir gently to combine.
5. Cover and refrigerate for about 1 hour.

Estimated nutrients per serving:
Calories: 50
Total protein (grams): 1
Soy protein (grams): 0
Total carbohydrate (grams): 9
Total fat (grams): 1
Total fiber (grams): 3
Total fruit and vegetable (servings): 1

For prostate protection: *You can use this recipe as is.*

PICKLED CUCUMBER AND ONION

This is a modification of a recipe Rita's grandmother used to make in the summertime. It keeps for as long as a week in the refrigerator. Most of the marinade is drained off and only the flavor remains.

YIELD: 6 SERVINGS
PREPARATION TIME: 10 MINUTES, PLUS 4 HOURS' CHILLING TIME
COOKING TIME: 5 MINUTES

INGREDIENTS:
1 medium cucumber, thinly sliced
2 thin slices onion, separated into rings
½ cup vinegar
½ cup apple juice concentrate
2 tablespoons sugar

1. Layer cucumber and onion slices in heatproof bowl.
2. In a small saucepan, bring vinegar, apple juice, and sugar to a boil. Boil for 2 minutes.

3. Pour over cucumber and onion. Let cool.
4. Transfer to a jar, cover, and refrigerate for at least 4 hours.
5. Drain before serving.

Estimated nutrients per serving:
  Calories: 25
  Total protein (grams): 0
  Soy protein (grams): 0
  Total carbohydrate (grams): 6
  Total fat (grams): 0
  Total fiber (grams): 2
  Total fruit and vegetable (servings): 1

For prostate protection: *You can use this recipe as is.*

VIETNAMESE SALAD ROLLS

YIELD: 2 SERVINGS, 2 ROLLS EACH
PREPARATION TIME: 30 MINUTES
COOKING TIME: NONE

INGREDIENTS:
  2 cups shredded lettuce
  1 cup mung bean sprouts, coarsely chopped, blanched
  ¼ cup shredded carrot
  ¼ cup chopped cilantro leaves
  1 tablespoon crunchy peanut butter
  1 tablespoon boiling water
  ¼ teaspoon honey
  1 tablespoon rice vinegar
  1 teaspoon tamari soy sauce
  ⅛ teaspoon sesame oil
  ⅛ teaspoon red pepper flakes
  4 spring roll wrappers

1. In a medium bowl, combine lettuce, sprouts, carrot, and cilantro.
2. In a small bowl or teacup, combine peanut butter, boiling water,

honey, rice vinegar, soy sauce, sesame oil, and red pepper flakes. Add to vegetables. Stir gently to combine. Let sit for 5 minutes.

3. Soften spring roll wrappers in water. When soft, put one wrapper on a flat surface covered with a paper towel. Blot the top side of the wrapper with another paper towel. With a slotted spoon, lift one-fourth of the vegetable mixture from the bowl and place on one end of the wrapper to form a "log." Fold the sides of the wrapper toward the middle, then roll tightly to enclose the filling. Repeat with remaining ingredients.

Estimated nutrients per serving:
Calories: 130
Total protein (grams): 5
Soy protein (grams): 0
Total carbohydrate (grams): 19
Total fat (grams): 4.5
Total fiber (grams): 1.5
Total fruit and vegetable (servings): 2

For prostate protection: *For minimal dietary fat, omit peanut butter.*

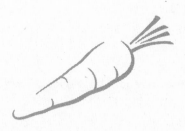

NEW AMERICAN

FRESH SPINACH AND RED CABBAGE SALAD

YIELD: 2 SERVINGS
PREPARATION TIME: 10 MINUTES
COOKING TIME: NONE

INGREDIENTS:

1 cup baby spinach leaves, bite-size pieces
½ cup finely shredded red cabbage
½ cup chopped baby bok choy
¼ medium Fuji apple, diced
3 tablespoons Tangy Tofu Dressing (page 201)

1. Place all vegetables and the apple in a salad bowl.
2. Add dressing; toss gently.

Estimated nutrients per serving:

Calories: 25
Total protein (grams): .5
Soy protein (grams): 0
Total carbohydrate (grams): 4
Total fat (grams): 1
Total fiber (grams): 1
Total fruit and vegetable (servings): 1½, including 1 serving of cruciferous
   vegetable

For prostate protection: You can use this recipe as is.

GARDEN SALAD

YIELD: 2 SERVINGS
PREPARATION TIME: 10 MINUTES
COOKING TIME: NONE

INGREDIENTS:

   ½ cup bite-size pieces romaine lettuce
   ½ cup bite-size pieces butter lettuce
   ½ cup shredded red cabbage
   ½ cup shredded green cabbage
   1 tablespoon Balsamic Vinegar Dressing (page 200)
   ½ cup fresh green soybeans

1. Place all vegetables in a salad bowl.
2. Add dressing; toss gently.
3. Add soybeans and toss again.

Estimated nutrients per serving:
   Calories: 100
   Total protein (grams): 6
   Soy protein (grams): 6
   Total carbohydrate (grams): 6
   Total fat (grams): 8
   Total fiber (grams): 3
   Total fruit and vegetable (servings): 1½, including 1 serving of cruciferous
      vegetable

For prostate protection: *You can use this recipe as is.*

HEALTHY COLESLAW

Rita brings this coleslaw to family picnics and it is always a hit. She said, "I bring huge bowls full, and they always eat it. The secret is just a tiny bit of sugar." This adaptation of her recipe has just ¼ teaspoon of sugar for 4 servings. The flavors develop if this is made several hours ahead of time and refrigerated.

YIELD: 4 SERVINGS
PREPARATION TIME: 15 MINUTES
COOKING TIME: NONE

INGREDIENTS:

   2 cups finely shredded cabbage
   1 large carrot, peeled and shredded

½ cup plain nonfat yogurt
¼ cup sweet pickle relish or chopped sweet pickle
1 tablespoon pickle juice
¼ teaspoon sugar

1. In a large bowl, combine cabbage and carrot.
2. To make dressing, combine yogurt, pickle, pickle juice, and sugar in a small bowl.
3. Pour dressing over vegetables and stir to combine.

Estimated nutrients per serving:
Calories: 60
Total protein (grams): 3
Soy protein (grams): 0
Total carbohydrate (grams): 12
Total fat (grams): 0
Total fiber (grams): 2
Total fruit and vegetable (servings): 1, including 1 serving of cruciferous vegetable

For prostate protection: To eliminate animal products, use silken tofu instead of nonfat yogurt.

MIXED GREENS AND TOMATO SALAD

YIELD: 2 SERVINGS
PREPARATION TIME: 10 MINUTES
COOKING TIME: NONE

INGREDIENTS:
1 cup bite-size pieces butter lettuce
1 cup bite-size pieces green leaf lettuce
½ cup chopped baby bok choy
¼ cup coarsely chopped parsley
1 small tomato, chopped
1 tablespoon Balsamic Vinegar Dressing (page 200)

1. Place all vegetables in a salad bowl.
2. Add dressing; toss gently.

Estimated nutrients per serving:
Calories: 50
Total protein (grams): 1
Soy protein (grams): 0
Total carbohydrate (grams): 5
Total fat (grams): 3
Total fiber (grams): 2
Total fruit and vegetable (servings): 2, including ½ serving of cruciferous vegetable

For prostate protection: *You can use this recipe as is.*

SPINACH AND ORANGE SALAD

This is wonderfully refreshing. The fruit is a nice addition to a spinach salad.

YIELD: 2 SERVINGS
PREPARATION TIME: 10 MINUTES
COOKING TIME: NONE

INGREDIENTS
2 cups bite-size pieces baby spinach leaves
1 small orange, peeled and sliced
1 slice red onion
2 tablespoons Balsamic Vinegar Dressing (page 200)

1. Combine spinach, orange, and onion in a bowl.
2. Add dressing, toss gently.

Estimated nutrients per serving:
Calories: 80
Total protein (grams): 2
Soy protein (grams): 0
Total carbohydrate (grams): 8
Total fat (grams): 6
Total fiber (grams): 2
Total fruit and vegetable (servings): 1½

For prostate protection: *You can use this recipe as is.*

SPRING GREENS

YIELD: 2 SERVINGS
PREPARATION TIME: 10 MINUTES
COOKING TIME: NONE

INGREDIENTS:

10 medium asparagus spears, stems trimmed, sliced on diagonal
10 small snow peas, ends trimmed, sliced on diagonal
2 cups bite-size pieces baby spinach leaves
1 tablespoon Balsamic Vinegar Dressing (page 200)

1. Blanch asparagus and peas separately.
2. Place all vegetables in a salad bowl.
3. Add dressing; toss gently.

Estimated nutrients per serving:

Calories: 45
Total protein (grams): 2
Soy protein (grams): 0
Total carbohydrate (grams): 3
Total fat (grams): 3
Total fiber (grams): 2
Total fruit and vegetable (servings): 2

For prostate protection: *You can use this recipe as is.*

GREEN SALAD

YIELD: 2 SERVINGS
PREPARATION TIME: 10 MINUTES
COOKING TIME: NONE

INGREDIENTS:

½ cup broccoli florets
½ cup bite-size pieces butter lettuce
½ cup bite-size pieces green leaf lettuce

½ *cup chopped baby bok choy*
2 *tablespoons Balsamic Vinegar Dressing (page 200)*

1. Blanch broccoli florets.
2. Place all vegetables in a salad bowl.
3. Add dressing; toss gently.

Estimated nutrients per serving:
Calories: 60
Total protein (grams): 1
Soy protein (grams): 0
Total carbohydrate (grams): 3
Total fat (grams): 6
Total fiber (grams): 1
Total fruit and vegetable (servings): 1½, including 1 serving of cruciferous
vegetable

For prostate protection: *You can use this recipe as is.*

MEDITERRANEAN

ROMA TOMATOES WITH OLIVE OIL

This is a delicous and very refreshing side salad. The fresh oregano leaves add a wonderful aroma to the peppered tomatoes. It is a perfect side salad for a warm, sunny summer day.

YIELD: 2 SERVINGS

PREPARATION TIME: 10 MINUTES

COOKING TIME: NONE

INGREDIENTS:

2 medium Roma tomatoes, sliced
1 teaspoon extra-virgin olive oil
1 teaspoon chopped fresh oregano leaves
Generous sprinkle freshly ground pepper

1. Arrange tomato slices on 2 individual serving plates.
2. Drizzle olive oil over the tomatoes.
3. Sprinkle with oregano and pepper.

Estimated nutrients per serving:

Calories: 30
Total protein (grams): 0
Soy protein (grams): 0
Total carbohydrate (grams): 2
Total fat (grams): 2
Total fiber (grams): 0
Total fruit and vegetable (servings): 1

For prostate protection: *For minimal dietary fat, use ½ instead of 1 teaspoon olive oil.*

BROCCOLI SALAD

You can use a potato peeler to make the slivers of jicama for this salad, which combines different textures, flavors, colors, and shapes.

YIELD: 2 SERVINGS
PREPARATION TIME: 15 MINUTES
COOKING TIME: NONE

INGREDIENTS:

1 cup broccoli florets, blanched
1 thin slice red onion, separated into rings
¼ cup slivered peeled jicama
2 tablespoons Lemon Dressing (page 201)

1. Place all vegetables in a salad bowl.
2. Add dressing; toss gently.

Estimated nutrients per serving:

Calories: 70
Total protein (grams): 2
Soy protein (grams): 0
Total carbohydrate (grams): 4
Total fat (grams): 6
Total fiber (grams): 2
Total fruit and vegetable (servings): 1, including 1 serving of cruciferous vegetable

For prostate protection: *You can use this recipe as is.*

MARINATED CAULIFLOWER

YIELD: 2 SERVINGS
PREPARATION TIME: 10 MINUTES
COOKING TIME: 5 MINUTES

INGREDIENTS:

¼ cup Lemon Dressing (page 201)
¼ teaspoon oregano

½ teaspoon chopped Italian parsley
1 cup small cauliflower florets

1. In a small bowl, combine Lemon Dressing, oregano, and parsley. Set aside.
2. Blanch cauliflower. Drain but do not rinse.
3. Immediately add to the dressing mixture. Stir gently to combine.
4. Let cool, cover, and refrigerate for at least 4 hours or overnight.
5. Drain before using.

Estimated nutrients per serving:
Calories: 40
Total protein (grams): 1
Soy protein (grams): 0
Total carbohydrate (grams): 3
Total fat (grams): 3
Total fiber (grams): 1
Total fruit and vegetable (servings): 1, including 1 serving of cruciferous vegetable

For prostate protection: *You can use this recipe as is.*

FIELD GREENS

This salad includes dandelion greens, which are now available in many large supermarkets and are a nice change from traditional salad greens.

YIELD: 2 SERVINGS
PREPARATION TIME: 10 MINUTES
COOKING TIME: NONE

INGREDIENTS:
12 small asparagus spears, cut in 1-inch diagonal slices and
    blanched
1 cup bite-size pieces dandelion greens
½ cup watercress leaves
¼ cup chopped celery
1½ tablespoons Balsamic Vinegar Dressing (page 200)

1. Place all vegetables in a salad bowl.
2. Add dressing; toss gently.

Estimated nutrients per serving:

Calories: 70
Total protein (grams): 3
Soy protein (grams): 0
Total carbohydrate (grams): 6
Total fat (grams): 4
Total fiber (grams): 2
Total fruit and vegetable (servings): 2

For prostate protection: *You can use this recipe as is.*

SPINACH AND GRATED-CARROT SALAD

YIELD: 2 SERVINGS
PREPARATION TIME: 10 MINUTES
COOKING TIME: NONE

INGREDIENTS:

2 cups bite-size pieces baby spinach leaves
1 small carrot, peeled and grated
1 small green onion, sliced
1 small radish, thinly sliced
1 teaspoon chopped fresh sweet marjoram leaves
2 tablespoons Balsamic Vinegar Dressing (page 200)

1. Combine all vegetables and the marjoram in a salad bowl.
2. Add dressing; toss gently.

Estimated nutrients per serving:

Calories: 70
Total protein (grams): 1
Soy protein (grams): 0
Total carbohydrate (grams): 4
Total fat (grams): 6
Total fiber (grams): 2
Total fruit and vegetable (servings): 2

For prostate protection: *You can use this recipe as is.*

SALAD WITH CAPERS

YIELD: 2 SERVINGS
PREPARATION TIME: 10 MINUTES
COOKING TIME: NONE

INGREDIENTS:

½ cup bite-size pieces romaine lettuce
½ cup bite-size pieces red leaf lettuce
1 cup shredded green cabbage
1 small tomato, chopped
½ tablespoon capers, chopped
1 tablespoon Lemon Dressing (page 201)

1. Place all vegetables in a salad bowl.
2. Add capers and dressing; toss.

Estimated nutrients per serving:

Calories: 50
Total protein (grams): 1
Soy protein (grams): 0
Total carbohydrate (grams): 5
Total fat (grams): 3
Total fiber (grams): 2
Total fruit and vegetable (servings): 2, including 1 serving of cruciferous vegetable

For prostate protection: *You can use this recipe as is.*

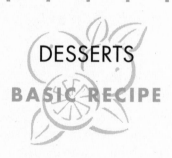

DESSERTS
BASIC RECIPE

COCONUT MILK

Superfine coconut is steeped in nonfat milk to produce a nonfat version of the traditional high-fat coconut milk. Use it in recipes as directed.

YIELD: 1 CUP
PREPARATION TIME: 5 MINUTES
COOKING TIME: 20 MINUTES

INGREDIENTS:
  1⅓ cups nonfat milk
  ⅔ cup superfine coconut

1. In a small saucepan, combine milk and coconut. Slowly bring to a boil.
2. Remove from heat immediately and let steep for 20 minutes.
3. Strain milk and discard coconut. Cover and refrigerate until cold. Strain through a fine sieve to remove any fat that has risen to the top.
4. Store in the refrigerator for as long as 5 days.

Estimated nutrients per cup:
  Calories: 90
  Total protein (grams): 8
  Soy protein (grams): 0
  Total carbohydrate (grams): 14
  Total fat (grams): 0
  Total fiber (grams): 0

For prostate protection: *To eliminate animal products, make coconut milk with water instead of nonfat milk.*

ASIAN

ORANGE SLICES IN ORANGE WATER

A hint of orange-blossom water transforms everyday oranges into an exotic dessert. This is quick and easy to prepare and very refreshing on a hot day.

YIELD: 2 SERVINGS
PREPARATION TIME: 5 MINUTES
COOKING TIME: NONE

INGREDIENTS:
½ cup water
½ teaspoon orange-blossom water
2 drops almond extract
¼ teaspoon vanilla extract
¼ teaspoon honey
Sprinkle cinnamon
2 oranges, peeled and sliced
2 sprigs fresh mint

1. In a small bowl, combine water, orange water, almond and vanilla extracts, honey, and cinnamon.
2. Pour over orange slices. Let sit for at least 20 minutes to blend flavors.
3. Serve topped with mint sprigs.

Estimated nutrients per serving:
Calories: 60
Total protein (grams): 1
Soy protein (grams): 0
Total carbohydrate (grams): 16
Total fat (grams): 0
Total fiber (grams): 3
Total fruit and vegetable (servings): 1

For prostate protection: *You can use this recipe as is.*

FRUIT JUMBLE

This combination of sweet-tangy fruits is a true pleasure to the palate.

YIELD: 2 SERVINGS
PREPARATION TIME: 10 MINUTES
COOKING TIME: NONE

INGREDIENTS:
   1 cup fresh or canned pineapple chunks
   1 cup fresh or canned mandarin orange sections
   6 canned lychees, halved
   ¼ cup liquid from canned lychees
   6 fresh raspberries

1. In a medium bowl, combine pineapple, orange sections, and lychees. Stir gently to mix.
2. Add lychee liquid and stir gently again.
3. Serve chilled topped with fresh raspberries.

Estimated nutrients per serving:
   Calories: 110
   Total protein (grams): 1
   Soy protein (grams): 0
   Total carbohydrate (grams): 27
   Total fat (grams): 1
   Total fiber (grams): 4
   Total fruit and vegetable (servings): 2½

For prostate protection: *You can use this recipe as is.*

GUAVA ICE

This ice is made using a small ice-cream maker with a cylinder that you freeze ahead of time for at least 8 hours. Actual preparation involves only an occasional turn of the handle, which will keep the ice at the right consistency for about an hour.

YIELD: 2 SERVINGS

PREPARATION TIME: 10 MINUTES, PLUS 20 MINUTES' FREEZING TIME

COOKING TIME: NONE

INGREDIENTS:

1 cup guava nectar
½ medium banana, cut in chunks
1 tablespoon toasted pistachio nuts

1. In a blender container, blend the guava nectar and banana.
2. Pour into frozen cylinder of ice-cream maker. Turn the handle every few minutes as indicated in the instruction booklet of the ice-cream maker.
3. Keep the guava-banana ice frozen in the cylinder and turn the handle every few minutes during the meal.
4. Top with pistachio nuts and serve immediately.

Estimated nutrients per serving:
Calories: 130
Total protein (grams): 1.5
Soy protein (grams): 0
Total carbohydrate (grams): 27
Total fat (grams): 2
Total fiber (grams): 2
Total fruit and vegetable (servings): 1

For prostate protection: *For minimal dietary fat, sprinkle with chopped crystallized ginger instead of pistachio nuts.*

MINTED MELON

In the summertime, when an expansive array of melons is available, try different melons as they reach their prime.

YIELD: 2 SERVINGS

PREPARATION TIME: 15 MINUTES, PLUS 1 HOUR OF CHILLING TIME

COOKING TIME: 30 MINUTES, TO REDUCE THE GINGER ALE

INGREDIENTS:

¼ *medium cantaloupe*
¼ *medium golden honeydew melon*
¼ *medium Persian melon*
10 *ounces ginger ale*
½ *tablespoon lightly packed chopped fresh mint*
2 *sprigs fresh mint*

1. Peel melons and cut in chunks. Place in a large bowl.
2. Put ginger ale in a medium saucepan and bring to a boil. Do not cover. Continue to boil gently until volume is reduced to about 4 ounces.
3. Add chopped mint to hot liquid. Remove from heat and let cool completely.
4. Pour over melon. Stir gently. Refrigerate for at least 1 hour.
5. Serve topped with mint sprigs.

Estimated nutrients per serving:

Calories: 100
Total protein (grams): 2
Soy protein (grams): 0
Total carbohydrate (grams): 26
Total fat (grams): 1
Total fiber (grams): 2
Total fruit and vegetable (servings): 1½

For prostate protection: *You can use this recipe as is.*

LYCHEE TAPIOCA

When served in a glass dish, this is a really pretty dessert. The colorful fruit is suspended in the translucent soft tapioca pudding. It is light and refreshing. Serve chilled, but don't keep for more than a day, as the tapioca becomes a thin liquid.

YIELD: 2 SERVINGS

PREPARATION TIME: 10 MINUTES, PLUS 1 HOUR OF CHILLING TIME

COOKING TIME: 5 MINUTES

INGREDIENTS:

¾ cup juice from canned lychees
¼ cup water
1 tablespoon minute tapioca
⅛ teaspoon ground ginger
1 (11-ounce) can mandarin oranges, drained
12 canned lychees, sliced
1 medium kiwifruit, peeled and diced

1. In a small saucepan, combine lychee juice and water. Stir in tapioca. Let sit for five minutes.
2. Cook over medium heat, stirring constantly, until mixture boils, about 5 minutes.
3. Remove from heat. Stir in ginger. Let cool.
4. Put mandarin oranges and lychee slices into serving dishes.
5. Pour tapioca mixture over fruit. Cover and refrigerate at least 1 hour or until well chilled.
6. Serve topped with kiwifruit.

Estimated nutrients per serving:
Calories: 140
Total protein (grams): 2
Soy protein (grams): 0
Total carbohydrate (grams): 34
Total fat (grams): 1
Total fiber (grams): 4
Total fruit and vegetable (servings): 1½

For prostate protection: *You can use this recipe as is.*

LYCHEES AND MANGO ICE

As with all ice recipes, you will need a small ice-cream maker with a cylinder that you freeze in advance (at least 8 hours). Preparation involves only an occasional turn of the handle so you can make it while you put together the rest of the meal. If you continue to turn every few minutes during the meal, the mango ice will maintain the right consistency for about an hour.

YIELD: 2 SERVINGS

PREPARATION TIME: 5 MINUTES, PLUS 20 MINUTES' FREEZING TIME

COOKING TIME: NONE

INGREDIENTS:

1½ cups mango nectar
1 teaspoon fresh lemon juice
12 fresh or canned lychees
2 sprigs fresh mint

1. Combine mango nectar and lemon juice.
2. Pour mixture into frozen cylinder of ice-cream maker. Turn the handle every few minutes as indicated in the instruction booklet.
3. Keep the mango ice frozen in the cylinder and turn the handle every few minutes during the meal.
4. Put into serving bowls. Add lychees. Garnish with mint sprigs.

Estimated nutrients per serving:

Calories: 140
Total protein (grams): 1
Soy protein (grams): 0
Total carbohydrate (grams): 33
Total fat (grams): 0.5
Total fiber (grams): 1.5
Total fruit and vegetable (servings): 2

For prostate protection: *You can use this recipe as is.*

BAKED BANANA IN ORANGE WATER

We created this recipe for Barbara, who loves fried bananas and wanted a lower-fat alternative that tasted great and completed the meal.

YIELD: 2 SERVINGS

PREPARATION TIME: 5 MINUTES

COOKING TIME: 20 MINUTES

INGREDIENTS:

2 small bananas, peeled and cut in half lengthwise
½ cup orange juice
¼ teaspoon honey
⅛ teaspoon orange-blossom water
1 teaspoon toasted sesame seeds

Preheat oven to 350 degrees.

1. Put the bananas, cut side up, in a glass or ceramic baking dish.
2. In a small bowl or teacup, combine orange juice, honey, and orange water.
3. Pour mixture over bananas.
4. Bake, covered, in preheated oven for 20 minutes.
5. Serve warm in the cooking liquid, topped with sesame seeds.

Estimated nutrients per serving:

Calories: 130
Total protein (grams): 2
Soy protein (grams): 0
Total carbohydrate (grams): 31
Total fat (grams): 1.5
Total fiber (grams): 2.5
Total fruit and vegetable (servings): 1½

For prostate protection: *For minimal dietary fat, omit sesame seeds.*

MANGO SORBET

Unlike recipes for other ices, this recipe does not use fruit puree but chunks of mango with mango nectar. You'll need a small ice-cream maker with a cylinder that you freeze in advance (at least 8 hours). Preparation involves only an occasional turn of the handle, so you can make it while you put together the rest of the meal. An occasional turn during the meal will keep the mango ice at the right consistency for about an hour.

YIELD: 2 SERVINGS

PREPARATION TIME: 5 MINUTES, PLUS 20 MINUTES'
FREEZING TIME

COOKING TIME: NONE

INGREDIENTS:

½ cup chopped fresh mango
1 cup mango nectar
1 teaspoon fresh lemon juice
2 slices fresh lemon
2 large strawberries

1. In a medium bowl, stir together the chopped mango and mango nectar. Stir in lemon juice.
2. Pour into frozen cylinder of ice-cream maker. Turn the handle every few minutes as indicated in the instruction booklet of the ice-cream maker.
3. Keep the sorbet frozen in the cylinder and turn the handle every few minutes during the meal.
4. Spoon into serving bowls. Decorate with lemon slices and strawberries.

Estimated nutrients per serving:

Calories: 100
Total protein (grams): 0.5
Soy protein (grams): 0
Total carbohydrate (grams): 25
Total fat (grams): 0
Total fiber (grams): 1.5
Total fruit and vegetable (servings): 1

For prostate protection: *You can use this recipe as is.*

MANGO LASSI

This popular Southeast Asian beverage makes a great light dessert. It's a perfect accompaniment to the spices in a curry. It can be made ahead of time and stored in the refrigerator until ready to serve.

YIELD: 2 SERVINGS

PREPARATION TIME: 5 MINUTES

COOKING TIME: NONE

INGREDIENTS:

2 cups plain nonfat yogurt
1 cup chopped fresh mango
½ cup mango nectar

1. Put all ingredients into a blender container.
2. Process on low until mango is pureed.
3. Pour into 2 glasses.

Estimated nutrients per serving:
Calories: 230
Total protein (grams): 14
Soy protein (grams): 0
Total carbohydrate (grams): 44
Total fat (grams): 1
Total fiber (grams): 1
Total fruit and vegetable (servings): 1

For prostate protection: *This recipe cannot be modified to meet the prostate cancer recommendations.*

COCONUT FLOAT

Don't be put off by the thought of making a gelatin dessert. This variation of the traditional almond float is easy to make and has a delightful flavor.

YIELD: 2 SERVINGS
PREPARATION TIME: 10 MINUTES, PLUS 2 HOURS
TO CHILL AND SET
COOKING TIME: NONE

INGREDIENTS:

1 envelope unflavored gelatin
½ cup cold water
½ cup boiling water
1 cup coconut milk (page 221)
⅛ teaspoon almond extract

1 medium kiwifruit, peeled and sliced
½ cup mandarin orange sections

1. In a medium bowl, combine the gelatin and cold water; let stand for 5 minutes.
2. Add boiling water; stir until gelatin is dissolved. Stir in coconut milk and almond extract.
3. Pour into 2 serving dishes. Cover and refrigerate until gelatin is set.
4. Top with kiwifruit slices and mandarin sections.

Estimated nutrients per serving:
Calories: 100
Total protein (grams): 8
Soy protein (grams): 0
Total carbohydrate (grams): 17
Total fat (grams): 0.5
Total fiber (grams): 2
Total fruit and vegetable (servings): 1

For prostate protection: *To eliminate animal products, make coconut milk with water instead of nonfat milk.*

MANDARIN AND BING CHERRY TAPIOCA

This tapioca combines two fruits very popular in many Asian cultures. We used fresh bing cherries. If fresh ones are not available, thaw frozen ones and drain them well to avoid "bleeding" and keep the tapioca clear. Serve chilled, but don't keep for more than a day, as the tapioca becomes a thin liquid.

YIELD: 2 SERVINGS
PREPARATION TIME: 10 MINUTES, PLUS 1 HOUR OF CHILLING TIME
COOKING TIME: 5 MINUTES

INGREDIENTS:
1 (11-ounce) can mandarin oranges
1 tablespoon minute tapioca

1 teaspoon corn syrup
⅛ teaspoon almond extract
8 medium fresh bing cherries, halved and seeded
2 mint sprigs

1. Drain the mandarin oranges, reserving juice. Put juice in a measuring cup and add water to make 1 cup.
2. Pour into small saucepan. Stir in tapioca. Let sit for 5 minutes.
3. Cook over medium heat, stirring constantly, until mixture boils, about 5 minutes.
4. Remove from heat. Stir in corn syrup and almond extract. Let cool.
5. Put orange sections and cherry halves into serving dishes.
6. Pour tapioca mixture over fruit. Cover and refrigerate at least 1 hour or until well chilled.
7. Serve garnished with mint sprigs.

Estimated nutrients per serving:
Calories: 110
Total protein (grams): 1
Soy protein (grams): 0
Total carbohydrate (grams): 27
Total fat (grams): 0.5
Total fiber (grams): 3
Total fruit and vegetable (servings): 1½

For prostate protection: You can use this recipe as is.

POACHED ASIAN PEARS

Asian pears are firm and crunchy even when ripe. They will retain some of their firmness when cooked. The pears are most flavorful when served hot.

YIELD: 2 SERVINGS

PREPARATION TIME: 5 MINUTES

COOKING TIME: 20 TO 30 MINUTES

INGREDIENTS:

2 *small Asian pears*
1 *tablespoon currants*
⅓ *cup water*
2 *drops vanilla extract*

Preheat oven to 350 degrees.

1. Cut pears in half lengthwise; remove stems and cores. Place in a small ovenproof dish, cut side up.
2. Fill core spaces with currants.
3. Put ⅓ cup water and vanilla in the baking dish. Cover and bake for 20 to 30 minutes, until of desired doneness.

Estimated nutrients per serving:

Calories: 110
Total protein (grams): 1
Soy protein (grams): 0
Total carbohydrate (grams): 29
Total fat (grams): 1
Total fiber (grams): 4
Total fruit and vegetable (servings): 1

For prostate protection: *You can use this recipe as is.*

NEW AMERICAN

LEMON-RASPBERRY SORBET

A small ice-cream maker with a cylinder that you freeze is needed for this and other frozen desserts in this book. Because the cylinder has to be completely frozen to prepare these desserts, freeze it for at least 8 hours in advance. The preparation of these recipes involves only an occasional turn of the handle, so you can make them while you put together the rest of the meal. An occasional turn during the meal will keep the sorbet the right consistency for about an hour. These frozen desserts do not retain their soft-ice texture when stored in the freezer for more than 2 hours.

YIELD: 2 SERVINGS
PREPARATION TIME: 5 MINUTES, PLUS 20
    MINUTES' FREEZING TIME
COOKING TIME: NONE

INGREDIENTS:
   1 cup lemonade
   ½ cup fresh or frozen raspberries

1. In a blender container, blend the lemonade and raspberries.
2. Pour into frozen cylinder of ice-cream maker. Turn the handle every few minutes as indicated in the instruction booklet of the ice-cream maker.
3. Keep the sorbet frozen in the cylinder and turn the handle every few minutes during the meal.
4. Serve immediately.

Estimated nutrients per serving:
   Calories: 80
   Total protein (grams): 1
   Soy protein (grams): 0
   Total carbohydrate (grams): 20
   Total fat (grams): 0.5

Total fiber (grams): 4

Total fruit and vegetable (servings): 1

For prostate protection: *You can use this recipe as is.*

OATMEAL COOKIES

These sweet and delicious cookies are a big hit with Rita's kids. Her grandson likes them with low-fat milk for an afternoon snack. They are perfect for those "sugar-craving" moments. Each cookie has 2 grams of soy protein.

YIELD: 20 COOKIES, 2 COOKIES PER SERVING

PREPARATION TIME: 15 MINUTES

COOKING TIME: 25 MINUTES

INGREDIENTS:

¾ cup soy flour

½ teaspoon baking powder

⅛ teaspoon cinnamon

1½ cups rolled oats

1 large egg

½ cup applesauce

½ cup raisins

½ cup brown sugar

¼ cup sugar

¼ cup extra-light olive oil

Preheat oven to 300 degrees.

1. Stir together flour, baking powder, and cinnamon. Add oats.
2. In another bowl, beat egg. Mix in applesauce, raisins, and sugars. Beat in olive oil until blended.
3. Make a well in the center of flour mixture. Pour in egg mixture; stir gently until just mixed. Do not beat.
4. Drop by heaping tablespoons onto cookie sheet that has been lightly brushed with extra-light olive oil. Flatten until dough is 2½ to 3 inches in diameter.
5. Bake in preheated oven for 25 minutes.

6. Remove from oven and cool on cookie sheet for 10 minutes, then transfer cookies to a cooling rack.

Estimated nutrients per serving:
Calories: 220
Total protein (grams): 6
Soy protein (grams): 4
Total carbohydrate (grams): 34
Total fat (grams): 7
Total fiber (grams): 3
Total fruit and vegetable (servings): none

For prostate protection: *This recipe cannot be modified to meet the prostate cancer recommendations.*

GINGER YOGURT

This refreshing dessert with two forms of ginger is great either by itself or with fruit.

YIELD: 2 SERVINGS
PREPARATION TIME: 5 MINUTES
COOKING TIME: NONE

INGREDIENTS:
1½ cups plain nonfat yogurt
1 tablespoon apple juice
1 teaspoon chopped crystallized ginger
½ teaspoon powdered ginger

Combine all ingredients.

Estimated nutrients per serving:
Calories: 110
Total protein (grams): 11
Soy protein (grams): 0
Total carbohydrate (grams): 15

Total fat (grams): 0
Total fiber (grams): 0
Total fruit and vegetable (servings): none

For prostate protection: *This recipe cannot be modified to meet the prostate cancer recommendations.*

FRESH FIGS AND WALNUTS
WITH VANILLA TOPPING

This delightful dessert is a way to take advantage of scrumptious fresh figs. Keep in mind that they spoil easily, so purchase ripe figs and use promptly.

YIELD: 2 SERVINGS
PREPARATION TIME: 10 MINUTES
COOKING TIME: NONE

INGREDIENTS:
  2 ounces Neufchâtel cheese (reduced-fat cream cheese)
  2 teaspoons nonfat soy milk
  ¼ teaspoon vanilla extract
  ½ teaspoon apple juice concentrate
  4 medium fresh figs
  1 tablespoon chopped toasted walnuts
  2 small mint sprigs

1. In a small bowl, whip the Neufchâtel cheese, soy milk, vanilla, and apple juice concentrate.
2. Wash figs gently, slice, and arrange on 2 serving plates.
3. Spoon topping over figs. Decorate with walnuts.
4. Garnish with mint sprigs.

Estimated nutrients per serving:
  Calories: 180
  Total protein (grams): 4
  Soy protein (grams): 0
  Total carbohydrate (grams): 22

Total fat (grams): 9
Total fiber (grams): 4
Total fruit and vegetable (servings): 1

For prostate protection: *This recipe cannot be modified to meet the prostate cancer recommendations.*

BAKED APPLES WITH VANILLA YOGURT

This is Barbara's favorite dessert, made with either naturally sweet-tart Fuji or tart Granny Smith apples. The combination of dried cranberries with the raisins and almonds adds pizzazz to this old-time favorite.

YIELD: 2 SERVINGS
PREPARATION TIME: 10 MINUTES
COOKING TIME: 1 HOUR

INGREDIENTS:
2 medium Fuji apples
1 tablespoon dried cranberries
1 tablespoon raisins
1 tablespoon slivered almonds, toasted
¼ cup apple juice
¼ cup nonfat vanilla yogurt

Preheat oven to 350 degrees.
1. Remove cores from apples; do not peel. Cut the skin around the "equator" of the apples to prevent them from bursting during cooking.
2. Put apples in an ovenproof dish. Combine cranberries, raisins, and nuts; place into the core space.
3. Pour apple juice over the apples.
4. Cover; bake on the lowest oven rack for 1 hour or until soft.
5. Serve warm topped with vanilla yogurt.

Estimated nutrients per serving:
Calories: 170
Total protein (grams): 3

Soy protein (grams): 0
Total carbohydrate (grams): 36
Total fat (grams): 3
Total fiber (grams): 6
Total fruit and vegetable (servings): 1

For prostate protection:
- *For minimal dietary fat, omit almonds.*
- *To eliminate animal products, omit yogurt.*

POACHED PEARS WITH NUTMEG TOPPING

These pears can bake in the oven with the entrée and be ready to serve warm as dessert. They are refreshing to the palate when served chilled.

YIELD: 2 SERVINGS
PREPARATION TIME: 15 MINUTES
COOKING TIME: 30 MINUTES

INGREDIENTS:
2 medium red Anjou pears
½ cup pear juice or red wine
⅛ teaspoon cinnamon
2 thin lemon slices
2 ounces Neufchâtel cheese (reduced-fat cream cheese)
2 teaspoons nonfat soy milk
⅛ teaspoon nutmeg
½ teaspoon pear juice

Preheat oven to 350 degrees.
1. Cut pears into quarters and remove the cores. Do not peel.
2. In a small casserole dish, combine the ½ cup pear juice or wine, cinnamon, and lemon slices.
3. Add pear quarters; baste with juice from the bottom of the dish.
4. Cover; bake in preheated oven for 20 to 30 minutes or until soft.
5. In a small bowl, whip the Neufchâtel cheese, soy milk, nutmeg, and ½ teaspoon pear juice.
6. Serve pears in their cooking liquid. Spoon topping over the pears.

Estimated nutrients per serving:

Calories: 200

Total protein (grams): 4

Soy protein (grams): 0

Total carbohydrate (grams): 32

Total fat (grams): 7

Total fiber (grams): 5

Total fruit and vegetable (servings): 1

For prostate protection: *To eliminate animal products, use silken tofu instead of Neufchâtel cheese for topping.*

CHOCOLATE PUDDING

To our surprise, it took many tries and Barbara's determination to succeed in having a soy-based chocolate pudding (her American "comfort food") in this book. The obvious modification was to use chocolate soy milk, which we tried first. We weren't pleased with the results. This version uses nonfat milk and soy protein powder. There are two important steps in this recipe. First is the *thorough* mixing of the dry ingredients to prevent lumping. Second is stirring *constantly* until the mixture thickens or comes to a boil.

YIELD: 2 SERVINGS

PREPARATION TIME: 10 MINUTES

COOKING TIME: 15 MINUTES

INGREDIENTS:

1½ *tablespoons cornstarch*

2 *tablespoons cocoa*

1 *tablespoon packed soy protein powder*

1 *tablespoon sugar*

1 *cup nonfat milk*

⅛ *teaspoon vanilla extract*

1. In a small saucepan, thoroughly mix the cornstarch, cocoa, soy protein powder, and sugar. Add 3 tablespoons of the milk and blend until smooth.

2. Gradually add the remaining milk and stir until smooth.
3. Cook over medium heat, stirring constantly, for 15 minutes or until mixture becomes thick or boils.
4. Remove from heat; stir in vanilla. Serve warm or chilled.

Estimated nutrients per serving:
Calories: 150
Total protein (grams): 9
Soy protein (grams): 4
Total carbohydrate (grams): 22
Total fat (grams): 1
Total fiber (grams): 2
Total fruit and vegetable (servings): none

For prostate protection: *This recipe cannot be modified to meet the prostate cancer recommendations.*

STRAWBERRY FROZEN DESSERT

This recipe uses a small ice-cream maker as described in the introduction to Lemon-Raspberry Sorbet, page 234.

YIELD: 2 SERVINGS
PREPARATION TIME: 5 MINUTES, PLUS 20 MINUTES TO FREEZE
COOKING TIME: NONE

INGREDIENTS:
¾ cup nonfat vanilla-flavored soy milk
¾ cup fresh or frozen strawberries

1. In a blender container, blend the soy milk and strawberries.
2. Pour into frozen cylinder of ice-cream maker. Turn the handle every few minutes as indicated in the instruction booklet of the ice-cream maker.
3. Keep the dessert frozen in the cylinder and turn the handle every few minutes during the meal.
4. Serve immediately.

Estimated nutrients per serving:
Calories: 70
Total protein (grams): 3
Soy protein (grams): 2
Total carbohydrate (grams): 14
Total fat (grams): 0
Total fiber (grams): 3
Total fruit and vegetable (servings): ½

For prostate protection: *You can use this recipe as is.*

TAPIOCA PUDDING

Tapioca pudding is an all-American "comfort food." Enjoy this recipe without guilt. We developed the recipe to be low in fat and include soy protein.

YIELD: 4 SERVINGS
PREPARATION TIME: 15 MINUTES
COOKING TIME: 20 MINUTES

INGREDIENTS:
3 tablespoons minute tapioca
1 tablespoon soy protein powder
3 tablespoons brown sugar
1 large egg
3 cups nonfat milk
⅛ teaspoon vanilla extract

1. In a medium saucepan, thoroughly mix the tapioca, soy protein powder, and brown sugar.
2. Beat the egg and milk together. Add ¼ cup of this mixture to the dry ingredients and blend until smooth.
3. Gradually add the remaining milk mixture and stir until smooth. Let stand 5 minutes.
4. Cook over medium heat, stirring constantly, for 20 minutes or until mixture comes to a full boil.
5. Remove from heat; stir in vanilla. Cool 20 minutes, stirring occasionally. Mixture thickens as it cools. Serve warm or chilled.

Estimated nutrients per serving:
  Calories: 160
  Total protein (grams): 10
  Soy protein (grams): 2
  Total carbohydrate (grams): 26
  Total fat (grams): 2
  Total fiber (grams): 0
  Total fruit and vegetable (servings): none

For prostate protection: *This recipe cannot be modified to meet the prostate cancer recommendations.*

FRUIT COMPOTE

Fruit compote is traditionally served warm as a wintertime dessert. When served chilled it is a refreshing summertime treat. It must be prepared ahead so the flavors can blend; it keeps well in the refrigerator for as long as 2 weeks.

YIELD: 4 SERVINGS
PREPARATION TIME: 10 MINUTES
COOKING TIME: NONE

INGREDIENTS:
  4 medium dried pear halves
  8 medium dried apple slices
  ½ cup dried cherries
  8 medium pitted prunes
  2 cups hot water
  ¼ teaspoon vanilla
  1/16 teaspoon cardamom powder
  1/16 teaspoon grated nutmeg

1. Cut pears and apples into big chunks.
2. Combine all fruits in a container with a lid.
3. Add hot water, vanilla, cardamom, and nutmeg.
4. Cover and refrigerate overnight.

Estimated nutrients per serving:

   Calories: 140
   Total protein (grams): 1
   Soy protein (grams): 0
   Total carbohydrate (grams): 36
   Total fat (grams): 0
   Total fiber (grams): 4
   Total fruit and vegetable (servings): 2

For prostate protection: *You can use this recipe as is.*

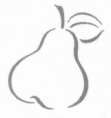

MEDITERRANEAN

MIXED BERRY ICE

This ice is made using a small ice-cream maker as described in the introduction to Lemon-Raspberry Sorbet, page 234.

It is extremely refreshing, delicious, and simple to make. It's also superhealthy, since it consists almost exclusively of berries, which are very high in antioxidants.

YIELD: 2 SERVINGS

PREPARATION TIME: 10 MINUTES, PLUS 20
    MINUTES' FREEZING TIME

COOKING TIME: NONE

INGREDIENTS:

1 cup mixed berries (raspberries, blueberries, blackberries, and
    strawberries)
1 tablespoon apple juice concentrate
½ cup water

1. In a blender container, blend the berries, apple juice concentrate, and water.
2. Pour into frozen cylinder of ice-cream maker. Turn the handle every few minutes as indicated in the instruction booklet of the ice-cream maker.
3. Keep the berry ice frozen in the cylinder and turn the handle every few minutes during the meal.
4. Serve immediately.

Estimated nutrients per serving:
    Calories: 50
    Total protein (grams): 0
    Soy protein (grams): 0
    Total carbohydrate (grams): 12
    Total fat (grams): 0

Total fiber (grams): 3
Total fruit and vegetable (servings): 1

For prostate protection: *You can use this recipe as is.*

MINTED MELON SLICES

This recipe combines three different melons having distinctive colors and flavors. Serve it often in the summer when melons are plentiful and inexpensive.

YIELD: 2 SERVINGS
PREPARATION TIME: 10 MINUTES
COOKING TIME: NONE

INGREDIENTS:
   ¼ small Persian melon, seeds and rind removed
   ⅛ small casaba melon, seeds and rind removed
   ¼ small honeydew melon, seeds and rind removed
   1 tablespoon chopped spearmint leaves
   2 large strawberries

1. Cut the melons into thin slices. Toss with mint leaves.
2. Arrange on 2 individual serving plates.
3. Garnish with strawberries.

Estimated nutrients per serving:
   Calories: 100
   Total protein (grams): 2
   Soy protein (grams): 0
   Total carbohydrate (grams): 26
   Total fat (grams): 0
   Total fiber (grams): 2
   Total fruit and vegetable (servings): 2

For prostate protection: *You can use this recipe as is.*

PLUMS WITH YOGURT

YIELD: 2 SERVINGS
PREPARATION TIME: 10 MINUTES
COOKING TIME: NONE

INGREDIENTS:
   3 large plums, each a different variety
   ½ cup nonfat vanilla yogurt
   1 teaspoon chopped roasted pistachio nuts

1. Cut the plums in half and remove the seeds. Slice.
2. Place plum slices in a bowl. Mix to distribute evenly.
3. Put into 2 individual serving bowls. Top with yogurt; sprinkle with pistachio nuts.

Estimated nutrients per serving:
   Calories: 140
   Total protein (grams): 4
   Soy protein (grams): 0
   Total carbohydrate (grams): 29
   Total fat (grams): 2
   Total fiber (grams): 3
   Total fruit and vegetable (servings): 1

For prostate protection: *You can use this recipe as is.*

CITRUS-SPRITZED STRAWBERRIES

This is a very refreshing dessert. It's so simple to prepare that it's perfect as a lunch dessert, or in the afternoon as a quick pick-me-up. The sparkling water makes the strawberries tingle in your mouth, and the mint imparts a fresh aftertaste.

YIELD: 2 SERVINGS
PREPARATION TIME: 10 MINUTES
COOKING TIME: NONE

INGREDIENTS:

8 *large strawberries, hulled and sliced*
½ *cup lime- or lemon-flavored sparkling water*
4 *small mint leaves, chopped*

1. Put strawberries in 2 individual serving dishes.
2. Add sparkling water; let sit for 10 minutes.
3. Sprinkle with mint leaves.

Estimated nutrients per serving:

Calories: 22
Total protein (grams): 0
Soy protein (grams): 0
Total carbohydrate (grams): 5
Total fat (grams): 0
Total fiber (grams): 2
Total fruit and vegetable (servings): 1

For prostate protection: *You can use this recipe as is.*

BARBARA'S ORANGE DESSERT

Barbara developed this recipe using memories of her childhood. Blood oranges, named for the deep red color of their flesh, are popular in the Mediterranean region. Kumquats are a kind of tiny orange with a tangy taste. They are eaten raw, peel and all.

YIELD: 2 SERVINGS
PREPARATION TIME: 15 MINUTES
COOKING TIME: NONE

INGREDIENTS:

1 *medium navel orange*
1 *medium blood orange*
½ *cup mandarin orange sections*
1 *medium kumquat, chopped*

1. Working over a bowl to collect the juices, cut the peel and pith from the navel and blood oranges. Cut into slices.

2. Place the orange slices and sections, as well as the juice, in a serving dish; stir to mix. Top with chopped kumquat.

3. As an alternative, layer the oranges in 2 parfait dishes, starting with navel, then blood, then mandarin oranges. Top with chopped kumquat.

Estimated nutrients per serving:
Calories: 90
Total protein (grams): 2
Soy protein (grams): 0
Total carbohydrate (grams): 22
Total fat (grams): 0
Total fiber (grams): 5
Total fruit and vegetable (servings): 1

For prostate protection: *You can use this recipe as is.*

MELON, RASPBERRY, AND CHERRY COCKTAIL

YIELD: 2 SERVINGS
PREPARATION TIME: 15 MINUTES
COOKING TIME: NONE

INGREDIENTS:
1 cup honeydew melon balls
½ cup raspberries
¾ cup pitted cherries
1 tablespoon toasted slivered almonds, chopped

1. Gently combine all fruit in a bowl.
2. Divide between 2 individual serving bowls. Sprinkle with almonds.

Estimated nutrients per serving:
Calories: 120
Total protein (grams): 2
Soy protein (grams): 0
Total carbohydrate (grams): 25
Total fat (grams): 3

Total fiber (grams): 6
Total fruit and vegetable (servings): 2

For prostate protection: *You can use this recipe as is.*

CHEESE TART WITH KIWI AND STRAWBERRIES

Rita's mom has a great recipe for a cheese pie, which was always a favorite. This is an adaptation of her recipe. It has a great taste and creamy texture, just like the original recipe. And it contains 5 grams of soy protein per serving.

YIELD: 6 SERVINGS
PREPARATION TIME: 30 MINUTES
COOKING TIME: 18 MINUTES

INGREDIENTS:
4 ladyfingers
8 ounces Neufchâtel cheese (reduced-fat cream cheese)
1 cup low-fat ricotta cheese
1 cup plain nonfat yogurt
4 tablespoons packed soy protein powder
2 large eggs
2 teaspoons sugar
¼ teaspoon vanilla
2 large kiwifruit, peeled and sliced
2 cups strawberries, hulled and sliced in half lengthwise

Preheat oven to 350 degrees.

1. Crumble the ladyfingers into coarse crumbs.
2. Spread evenly over the bottom of an 8-inch round pan with a removable base.
3. Combine cheeses, yogurt, soy protein powder, eggs, sugar, and vanilla in a food processor. Process until smooth and well blended.
4. Gently pour over crumbs in pan. Some of the crumbs will float into the cheese mixture.

5. Bake in a preheated oven for 18 minutes.
6. Remove from oven. Cool for 10 minutes. Cover and refrigerate until cold.
7. To serve, arrange kiwi slices and strawberry halves on the top of the tart.

Estimated nutrients per serving:
Calories: 290
Total protein (grams): 19
Soy protein (grams): 5
Total carbohydrate (grams): 22
Total fat (grams): 15
Total fiber (grams): 2
Total fruit and vegetable (servings): 1

For prostate protection: *You can use this recipe as is.*

INDEX

antioxidants, defined, 23
Antipasto, 175–76
Apples, Baked, with Vanilla Yogurt, 238–39
Aram, Breakfast, 86–87
Aram Sandwich, 118–19
Artichoke Frittata, 74–76
Artichoke Heart Salad, Spring, 170–71
Asian menu plans, 24–25
  breakfast, 29
  dinner, 31–32
  lunch, 30–31
  prostate protection and, 26
  soy protein shakes, 25–27
  stocking the pantry for, 27–28
Asparagus and Carrot in Oyster Sauce, 61–62
Asparagus and Radish Salad, 204–05
Asparagus Salad, Tuna-, 166–67

Bagel, Rye, with Savory Spread, 71–72
Baked Apples with Vanilla Yogurt, 238–39
Baked Banana in Orange Water, 227–28
Baked Beans, 144–45
Baked Roma Tomatoes with Fresh Basil, 198
Baked Trout Fillets, 163–64
Balsamic Vinegar Dressing, 200
Banana, Baked, in Orange Water, 227–28

Barbara's Orange Dessert, 248–49
barley, cooking instructions, 180–81
Barley Salad, Vegetable and, 176–77
Bars, Date Breakfast, 82–83
Basic White Sauce, 90
Bean and Broccoli Burrito with Tomato-Corn Salsa, 143–44
bean dishes
  Baked Beans, 144–45
  Bean and Broccoli Burrito with Tomato-Corn Salsa, 143–44
  Black Bean and Mushroom Stew with Parmesan Polenta, 98–99
  Black Bean and Rice Soup, 101–02
  Three-Bean Chili, 100–01
  Vegetable and Bean Ragout over Couscous, 106–07
  White Bean Stew, 104–05
beans. *See also* bean dishes; *the various soybeans*
  cooking instructions, 179–80, 181–82
Bean Sprout Salad, 205–06
Black Bean and Mushroom Stew with Parmesan Polenta, 98–99
Black Bean and Rice Soup, 101–02
Black Mushroom Soup, 92–93
Bok Choy, Wilted Baby, 195–96
Bok Choy and Tempeh, Sweet and Sour, 132–33
Bouillabaisse, 108–09
breads
  Corn Bread, 186–87

breads (*continued*)
lentil-nut loaf, 111–12
Olive Soda Bread, 84–85
Breakfast Aram, 86–87
Breakfast Bars, Date, 82–83
breakfast menu plans
Asian, 29
Mediterranean, 40–41
New American, 34–35
Breakfast Roll, Savory, 79–81
Breakfast Smoothie, Soy, 47–48
breast cancer
cruciferous vegetables and, 16–18
dietary protection against, 3–4, 9–10
flaxseed and, 15
insulin and, 18
prostate cancer risk and, 6
vitamin D and, 18
breast health
benefits of soy, 10–11
fruits and vegetables and, 19
Breast-Healthy Soy Protein Shake, 25–26
Broccoli, Curried Soybeans and, 136–37
Broccoli Burrito with Tomato-Corn
Salsa, Bean and, 143–44
Broccoli-Mushroom Stir-Fry with Tofu,
125–27
Broccoli Salad, 217
brown rice. *See individual rice dishes;*
rice, brown; rice accompaniments
Buckwheat Crepes with Date-Orange
Filling, 77–78
Buckwheat Pancakes with Berries, 66–67
bulgur, about, 39 n
bulgur dishes
English Chicken-Mushroom Casse-
role, 153–54
Green Cabbage Stuffed with Bulgur
and Vegetables, 156–57
Kubbul, 161–162
Spring Cracked Wheat Salad, 173–74

Cabbage, Sicilian, 199
Cabbage, Green, Stuffed with Bulgur
and Vegetables, 156–57
Cabbage Salad, Fresh Spinach and
Red, 210
Cake, Coffee, 72–73
cancer risk, shared among husbands and
wives, 6

Carrot Curry with Tofu, Cauliflower
and, 131–32
Carrot-Daikon Salad, 203
Carrot in Oyster Sauce, Asparagus and,
61–62
Carrot Salad, Spinach and Grated-, 219
Carrots and Collard Greens, Lemon,
197
Cauliflower, Marinated, 217–18
Cauliflower and Carrot Curry with Tofu,
131–32
Cauliflower and Fresh Soybeans,
Steamed, 196
Celery and Water Chestnut Salad,
206–07
cereals
Crunchy Homemade Granola, 67–69
fortified, 18
Homemade Muesli, 63–64
Steel-Cut Oatmeal with Sun-Dried
Cranberries and Walnuts, 64–65
Cheese, Macaroni and, 145–46
Cheese Tart with Kiwi and Strawberries,
250–51
Cherry Cocktail, Melon, Raspberry, and,
249–50
Cherry Tapioca, Mandarin and Bing,
231–32
Chicken, Sweet and Sour, 140–41
Chicken-Mushroom Casserole, English,
153–54
Chili, Three-Bean, 100–01
Chocolate Pudding, 240–41
Chutney, Fresh Papaya and Mango,
120–21
Chutney, Mint, 121–22
Citrus Delight, 85–86
Citrus-Spritzed Strawberries,
247–48
Coconut Float, 230–31
coconut milk, homemade, 221
Coffee Cake, 72–73
Coleslaw, Healthy, 211–12
Collard Greens, Lemon Carrots and,
197
collard greens, steamed, 192–93
conversion table, weight and measures,
22
Cookies, Oatmeal, 235–36
cooking terms, 21–22
Corn Bread, 186–87

Cornmeal Waffles with Peaches and
    Berries, 76–77
cost of stocking your pantry, 23
Cottage Pie, 149–50
Coucous with Dried Fruit and Almonds,
    81–82
couscous, about, 39n
Couscous, Vegetable and Bean Ragout
    over, 106–07
Cracked Wheat Salad, Spring, 173–74
Crepes, Buckwheat, with Date-Orange
    Filling, 77–78
Crispy Noodles with Vegetables, 56–57
cruciferous vegetables
    breast cancer and, 16–18
    supertasters and, 17
Crunchy Homemade Granola, 67–69
Cucumber and Onion, Pickled, 207–08
Cucumber Soup, Kale and, 97–98
Curried Soybeans and Broccoli,
    136–37
Curried Tofu, 52–53
Curry, Cauliflower and Carrot, with
    Tofu, 131–32
Custard, Enoki Mushroom, 54–55

Daikon Salad, Carrot-, 203
Date Breakfast Bars, 82–83
Date-Orange Muffins, 70–71
desserts. See also fruit dishes and
        desserts; ices, sorbets, and frozen
        dessert
    Cheese Tart with Kiwi and Strawber-
        ries, 250–51
    Chocolate Pudding, 240–41
    Coconut Float, 230–31
    Fresh Figs and Walnuts with Vanilla
        Topping, 237–38
    Ginger Yogurt, 236–37
    Lychee Tapioca, 225–26
    Mandarin and Bing Cherry Tapioca,
        231–32
    Mango Lassi, 229–30
    Oatmeal Cookies, 235–36
    Tapioca Pudding, 242–43
dinner menu plans
    Asian, 31–32
    Mediterranean, 42–43
    New American, 36–37
dressings. See salad dressings

Dried Fruit and Almonds, Couscous
    with, 81–82

eating plan, changing your, 20–21
edamame. See soybeans, fresh green
Egg Foo Yung, 58–59
Eggplant Salad, Roasted Peppers and,
    174–75
Eggs Florentine, 65–66
English Chicken-Mushroom Casserole,
    153–54
Enoki Mushroom Custard, 54–55
estrogen
    breast cancer and, 10, 16–17
    fiber and, 19
    genistein, 11
    "good" and "bad," 16–17
extra-light-taste olive oil, about, 39n
extra-virgin olive oil, about, 39n

Fajitas, 154–55
fats, about, 15–16
fiber, about, 19–20
Field Greens, 218–19
Figs, Goat Cheese with Melon and, 74
Figs, Fresh, and Walnuts with Vanilla
    Topping, 237–38
Fischler, Claude, 5
fish dishes
    Baked Trout Fillets, 163–64
    Fish with Carrot and Broccoli in
        Plum Sauce, 139–40
    Fried Rice with Shrimp, 184–85
    Grilled Fresh Tuna, 134–35
    Grilled Salmon with Sesame and
        Lime, 150–51
    Grilled Swordfish with Roasted Corn
        and Red Pepper Salsa, 146–47
    Laotian Fish Soup, 95–96
    Salmon Luncheon Salad, 171–72
    Swordfish Kebobs, 159
    Tuna-Asparagus Salad, 166–67
    Tuna Melt, 114–15
Fish with Carrot and Broccoli in Plum
    Sauce, 139–40
flax, potential benefits of, 15
fortified cereals, 18
Fresh Figs and Walnuts with Vanilla
    Topping, 237–38

Fresh Papaya and Mango Chutney, 120–21
Fresh Soybeans and Vegetables with Black Bean Sauce, 130–31
Fresh Spinach and Red Cabbage Salad, 210
Fresh Vegetable Medley, 194–95
Fried Rice with Shrimp, 184–85
Frittata, Artichoke, 74–76
frozen dessert. See ices, sorbets, and frozen dessert
Fruit Compote, 243–44
fruit dishes and desserts. See also ices, sorbets, and frozen dessert
    Baked Apples with Vanilla Yogurt, 238–39
    Baked Banana in Orange Water, 227–28
    Barbara's Orange Dessert, 248–49
    Citrus Delight, 85–86
    Citrus-Spritzed Strawberries, 247–48
    Fruit Compote, 243–44
    Fruit Jumble, 223
    Goat Cheese with Melon and Figs, 74
    Grilled Grapefruit Half, 83–84
    Melon, Raspberry, and Cherry Cocktail, 249–50
    Minted Melon, 224–25
    Minted Melon Slices, 246–47
    Orange Slices in Orange Water, 222
    Plums with Yogurt, 247
    Poached Asian Pears, 232–33
    Poached Pears with Nutmeg Topping, 239–40
Fruit Jumble, 223
fruits, health benefits of, 18–19

Garden Salad, 210–11
genistein (estrogen), 11
gingerroot, about, 28n
Ginger Yogurt, 236–37
Goat Cheese with Melon and Figs, 74
Goodwin, Pamela J., 18
grains. See also individual grains
    about whole, 18
Granola, Crunchy Homemade, 67–69
Grapefruit Half, Grilled, 83–84
gravy, vegetable, 89

Greek Sandwich, 117–18
Green Cabbage Stuffed with Bulgur and Vegetables, 156–57
greens. See salads, side
Green Salad, 214–15
Griddle Rice Cakes, 51–52
Grilled Fresh Tuna, 134–35
Grilled Grapefruit Half, 83–84
Grilled Marinated Mushrooms and Tomatoes, 57–58
Grilled Salmon with Sesame and Lime, 150–51
Grilled Swordfish with Roasted Corn and Red Pepper Salsa, 146–47
Guava Ice, 223–24

Healthy Coleslaw, 211–12
Homemade Muesli, 63–64
Hummus, Soybean, 182–83

ices, sorbets, and frozen dessert
    Guava Ice, 223–24
    Lemon-Raspberry Sorbet, 234–35
    Lychees and Mango Ice, 226–27
    Mango Sorbet, 228–29
    Mixed Berry Ice, 245–46
    Strawberry Frozen Dessert, 241–42
indole-3–carbinol, 18
    vegetables containing, 17
ingredients. See also individual ingredients
    cost of, 23
    shopping for, 23
    stocking, 27–28, 33–34, 39–40
insulin, breast cancer and, 18

kale, steamed, 192–93
Kale and Cucumber Soup, 97–98
Kale Pilaf, Rice and, 190
Kale Soup, Potato-, 105–06
Kebobs, Swordfish, 159
Kebobs, Tofu, 137–38
Kubbul, 161–62

Laotian Fish Soup, 95–96
Lasagna, 160–61
Lassi, Mango, 229–30

legumes. *See* bean dishes; beans; *lentil recipes; the various soybeans*
Lemon Carrots and Collard Greens, 197
Lemon Dressing, 201
Lemon-Raspberry Sorbet, 234–35
Lentil-Nut Loaf Sandwich, Open-Face, 111–12
lentils, cooking instructions, 179–80
Lentils, Linguini with, 157–58
Linguini with Lentils, 157–58
lunch menu plans
   Asian, 30–31
   Mediterranean, 41–42
   New American, 35–36
Lychees and Mango Ice, 226–27
Lychee Tapioca, 225–26

Macaroni and Cheese, 145–46
main-dish salads. *See* salads, main-dish
Mandarin and Bing Cherry Tapioca, 231–32
Mango Chutney, Fresh Papaya and, 120–21
Mango Ice, Lychees and, 226–27
Mango Lassi, 229–30
Mango Sorbet, 228–29
Marinated Cauliflower, 217–18
measures, conversion table, 22
Mediterranean menu plans, 37–38
   breakfast, 40–41
   dinner, 42–43
   lunch, 41–42
   prostate protection and, 38
   stocking the pantry for, 39–40
Melon, Minted, 224–25
Melon and Figs, Goat Cheese with, 74
Melon, Raspberry, and Cherry Cocktail, 249–50
Melon Slices, Minted, 246–47
menu plans. *See* Asian menu plans; Mediterranean menu plans; New American menu plans
Minestrone, 103–04
Mint Chutney, 121–22
Minted Melon, 224–25
Minted Melon Slices, 246–47
miso
   about, 13–14
   recipes using:
   Black Mushroom Soup, 92–93

Miso Soup, 53–54
Tofu-Mushroom Soup, 91–92
Miso Soup, 53–54
Mitchell, Rita, 4
Mixed Berry Ice, 245–46
Mixed-Grain Pilaf, 188–89
Mixed Greens and Tomato Salad, 212–13
Mixed Vegetable Stir-Fry, 123–124
Muesli, Homemade, 63–64
Muffins, Date-Orange, 70–71
mushroom dishes
   Black Bean and Mushroom Stew with Parmesan Polenta, 98–99
   Black Mushroom Soup, 92–93
   Broccoli-Mushroom Stir-Fry with Tofu, 125–27
   English Chicken-Mushroom Casserole, 153–54
   Enoki Mushroom Custard, 54–55
   Grilled Marinated Mushrooms and Tomatoes, 57–58
   Tofu-Mushroom Soup, 91–92
Mu Shu Vegetables, 124–25

New American menu plans, 32–33
   breakfast, 34–35
   dinner, 36–37
   lunch, 35–36
   prostate protection and, 33
   stocking the pantry for, 33–34
noodle dishes
   Asparagus and Carrot in Oyster Sauce, 61–62
   Crispy Noodles with Vegetables, 56–57
   Noodles with Celery, Carrots, and Broccoli, 141–42
   Rice Noodles with Vegetables and Tofu in Black Bean Sauce, 135–36
   Spicy Noodle Salad, 167–68
   Vegetable Pho, 50–51
   Vegetables and Tofu with Noodles, 128–29
Noodles with Celery, Carrot, and Broccoli, 141–42
nutrition information, 21

Oatmeal Cookies, 235–36
Oatmeal, Steel-Cut, with Sun-Dried Cranberries and Walnuts, 64–65

olive oil, about, 39n
Olive Soda Bread, 84–85
Onion, Pickled Cucumber and, 207–08
Open-Face Lentil-Nut Loaf Sandwich,
    111–12
Orange Dessert, Barbara's, 248–49
Orange Salad, Spinach and, 213
Orange Slices in Orange Water, 222
Orange Smoothie, Peach-, 78–79

Pancakes, Buckwheat, with Berries,
    66–67
pantry
    cost of stocking, 23
    stocking, 27–28, 33–34, 39–40
Papaya and Mango Chutney, Fresh,
    120–21
pasta dishes
    Lasagna, 160–61
    Linguini with Lentils, 157–58
    Macaroni and Cheese, 145–46
    Spaghetti with Tomato-Tempeh
        Sauce, 151–53
    Tricolor Pasta with Tomato and Soy-
        bean Sauce, 164–65
Peach-Orange Smoothie, 78–79
Pears, Poached, with Nutmeg Topping,
    239–40
Pears, Poached Asian, 232–33
Pepper, Stuffed Red, 148–49
Peppers, Roasted, and Eggplant Salad,
    174–75
Pho, Vegetable, 50–51
phytochemicals, defined, 23
Pickled Cucumber and Onion,
    207–08
Pie, Cottage, 149–50
Pilaf, Mixed-Grain, 188–89
Pilaf, Rice and Kale, 190
Pita Bread Sandwich, 116–17
Plums with Yogurt, 247
Poached Asian Pears, 232–33
Poached Pears with Nutmeg Topping,
    239–40
Polenta, Black Bean and Mushroom
    Stew with Parmesan, 98–99
Potato-Kale Soup, 105–06
Potato Salad, Vegetable-, 169–70
prostate cancer
    breast cancer risk and, 6

dietary protection against, 6, 26, 33,
    38
Prostate-Healthy Soy Protein Shake, 26–
    27
protein content of soy foods, 11
Pudding, Chocolate, 240–41
Pudding, Tapioca, 242–43

quinoa, cooking instructions, 187–88

Radish Salad, Asparagus and, 204–05
Ragout, Vegetable and Bean, over
    Couscous, 106–07
Raspberry Cocktail, Melon, Cherry, and,
    249–50
Raspberry Sorbet, Lemon-, 234–35
Ratatouille, 109–10
Red Pepper, Stuffed, 148–49
rice. See also individual rice dishes; rice
    accompaniments
    brown, cooking instructions, 178
    wild, cooking instructions, 179
Rice, Fried, with Shrimp, 184–85
rice accompaniments. See also individ-
    ual rice dishes
    Broccoli-Mushroom Stir-Fry with
        Tofu, 125–27
    Cauliflower and Carrot Curry with
        Tofu, 131–32
    Curried Soybeans and Broccoli,
        136–37
    Fish with Carrot and Broccoli in
        Plum Sauce, 139–40
    Fresh Soybeans and Vegetables with
        Black Bean Sauce, 130–31
    Fresh Vegetable Medley, 194–95
    Mixed Vegetable Stir-Fry, 123–24
    Spring Artichoke Heart Salad,
        170–71
    Sweet and Sour Bok Choy and Tem-
        peh, 132–33
    Sweet and Sour Chicken, 140–41
    Sweet and Sour Tofu, 127–28
    Tempeh with Snow Peas, Mushrooms,
        and Carrots, 49–50
    Tofu Kebobs, 137–38
Rice and Kale Pilaf, 190
Rice and Vegetables, 48
Rice Cakes, Griddle, 51–52

Rice Noodles with Vegetables and Tofu in Black Bean Sauce, 135–36
Rice Soup, Black Bean and, 101–02
Rice Vinegar Dressing, 202
Rice Wraps, 59–61
Roasted Peppers and Eggplant Salad, 174–75
Roll, Savory Breakfast, 79–81
Roma Tomatoes with Olive Oil, 216
Rye Bagel with Savory Spread, 71–72

salad dressings
  Balsamic Vinegar Dressing, 200
  Lemon Dressing, 201
  Rice Vinegar Dressing, 202
  Tangy Tofu Dressing, 201–02
salads, main-dish
  Antipasto, 175–76
  Roasted Peppers and Eggplant Salad, 174–75
  Salmon Luncheon Salad, 171–72
  Spicy Noodle Salad, 167–68
  Spring Artichoke Heart Salad, 170–71
  Spring Cracked Wheat Salad, 173–74
  Tuna-Asparagus Salad, 166–67
  Vegetable and Barley Salad, 176–77
  Vegetable-Potato Salad, 169–70
salads, side
  Asparagus and Radish Salad, 204–05
  Bean Sprout Salad, 205–06
  Broccoli Salad, 217
  Carrot-Daikon Salad, 203
  Celery and Water Chestnut Salad, 206–07
  Field Greens, 218–219
  Fresh Spinach and Red Cabbage Salad, 210
  Garden Salad, 210–11
  Green Salad, 214–15
  Healthy Coleslaw, 211–12
  Marinated Cauliflower, 217–18
  Mixed Greens and Tomato Salad, 212–13
  Pickled Cucumber and Onion, 207–08
  Roma Tomatoes with Olive Oil, 216
  Salad with Capers, 220
  Spinach and Grated-Carrot Salad, 219
  Spinach and Orange Salad, 213
  Spring Greens, 214

  Vietnamese Salad Rolls, 208–09
  Watercress Salad, 204
Salad with Capers, 220
Salmon, Grilled, with Sesame and Lime, 150–51
Salmon Luncheon Salad, 171–72
sandwiches. See also wraps
  Aram Sandwich, 118–19
  Greek Sandwich, 117–18
  Open-Face Lentil-Nut Loaf Sandwich, 111–12
  Pita Bread Sandwich, 116–17
  Smoked Tofu Sandwich, 112–13
  Tuna Melt, 114–15
sauce, white, 90
Sautéed Soybeans, 191
Savory Breakfast Roll, 79–81
Savory Spread, Rye Bagel with, 71–72
Shake, Breast-Healthy Soy Protein, 25–26
Shake, Prostate-Healthy Soy Protein, 26–27
shopping for ingredients, 23
Shrimp, Fried Rice with, 184–85
Sicilian Cabbage, 199
side salads. See salads, side
Smoked Tofu Sandwich, 112–13
Smoothie, Peach-Orange, 78–79
Smoothie, Soy Breakfast, 47–48
Soda Bread, Olive, 84–85
sorbet. See ices, sorbets, and frozen dessert
soups. See also stews
  Black Bean and Rice Soup, 101–02
  Black Mushroom Soup, 92–93
  Kale and Cucumber Soup, 97–98
  Laotian Fish Soup, 95–96
  Minestrone, 103–04
  Miso Soup, 53–54
  Potato-Kale Soup, 105–06
  Thai Soup, 93–94
  Tofu-Mushroom Soup, 91–92
soy. See also individual soy products; soy foods; the various soybeans
  breast benefits of, 10–11
  cautions regarding, 11–12
Soybean Hummus, 182–83
soybeans. See individual types
soybeans, fresh green
  about, 12

soybeans, fresh green (*continued*)
  recipes using:
  Crispy Noodles with Vegetables,
    56–57
  Fresh Soybeans and Vegetables with
    Black Bean Sauce, 130–31
  Fresh Vegetable Medley, 194–95
  Garden Salad, 210–11
  Laotian Fish Soup, 95–96
  Minestrone, 103–04
  Ratatouille, 109–10
  Salmon Luncheon Salad, 171–72
  Spring Cracked Wheat Salad, 173–74
  Steamed Cauliflower and Fresh Soy-
    beans, 196
  Thai Soup, 93–94
  Tricolor Pasta with Tomato and Soy-
    bean Sauce, 164–65
  Vegetable Pho, 50–51
soybeans, mature
  about, 12
  cooking instructions, 181–82
soybeans, mature or canned
  recipes using:
  Baked Beans, 144–45
  Curried Soybeans and Broccoli,
    136–37
  Green Cabbage Stuffed with Bulgur
    and Vegetables, 156–57
  Kubbul, 161–62
  Sautéed Soybeans, 191
  Soybean Hummus, 182–83
  Spring Artichoke Heart Salad, 170–71
  Three-Bean Chili, 100–01
  Vegetable and Barley Salad, 176–77
  Vegetable and Bean Ragout over
    Couscous, 106–07
  White Bean Stew, 104–05
soybeans, prepared black
  about, 12–13
  recipes using:
  Fish with Carrot and Broccoli in
    Plum Sauce, 139–40
  Fried Rice with Shrimp, 184–85
  Tuna-Asparagus Salad, 166–67
Soy Breakfast Smoothie, 47–48
soy flour
  about, 14
  recipes using:
  Coffee Cake, 72–73
  Corn Bread, 186–87

Oatmeal Cookies, 235–36
Olive Soda Bread, 84–85
soy foods. *See also individual soy
    products; soy; the various soybeans*
  protein content of, 11
soy milk
  about, 14
  recipes using:
  Buckwheat Pancakes with Berries,
    66–67
  Corn Bread, 186–87
  Cornmeal Waffles with Peaches and ·
    Berries, 76–77
  Crunchy Homemade Granola, 67–69
  Fresh Figs and Walnuts with Vanilla
    Topping, 237–38
  Macaroni and Cheese, 145–46
  Peach-Orange Smoothie, 78–79
  Poached Pears with Nutmeg Topping,
    239–40
  Prostate-Healthy Soy Protein Shake,
    26–27
  Rye Bagel with Savory Spread, 71–72
  Soy Breakfast Smoothie, 47–48
  Steel-Cut Oatmeal with Sun-Dried
    Cranberries and Walnuts, 64–65
  Strawberry Frozen Dessert, 241–42
soy protein powder
  about, 14
  recipes using:
  Aram Sandwich, 118–19
  Breast-Healthy Soy Protein Shake,
    25–26
  Buckwheat Pancakes with Berries,
    66–67
  Cheese Tart with Kiwi and Strawber-
    ries, 250–51
  Chocolate Pudding, 240–41
  Cornmeal Waffles with Peaches and
    Berries, 76–77
  Crunchy Homemade Granola,
    67–69
  Date Breakfast Bars, 82–83
  Date-Orange Muffins, 70–71
  Greek Sandwich, 117–18
  Homemade Muesli, 63–64
  Lasagna, 160–61
  Macaroni and Cheese, 145–46
  Prostate-Healthy Soy Protein Shake,
    26–27
  Rye Bagel with Savory Spread, 71–72

Savory Breakfast Roll, 79–81
Soy Breakfast Smoothie, 47–48
Steel-Cut Oatmeal with Sun-Dried
  Cranberries and Walnuts, 64–65
Tapioca Pudding, 242–43
Soy Protein Shake, Breast-Healthy,
  25–26
Soy Protein Shake, Prostate-Healthy,
  26–27
soy sauce, about, 14–15
soy tempeh. *See* tempeh
Spaghetti with Tomato-Tempeh Sauce,
  151–53
Spicy Noodle Salad, 167–68
Spinach and Grated-Carrot Salad, 219
Spinach and Orange Salad, 213
Spinach and Red Cabbage Salad, Fresh,
  210
Spring Artichoke Heart Salad, 170–71
Spring Cracked Wheat Salad, 173–74
Spring Greens, 214
Steamed Cauliflower and Fresh Soy-
  beans, 196
Steamed Collard Greens or Kale,
  192–93
Steel-Cut Oatmeal with Sun-Dried
  Cranberries and Walnuts, 64–65
stews. *See also* soups
  Black Bean and Mushroom Stew with
    Parmesan Polenta, 98–99
  Bouillabaisse, 108–09
  Ratatouille, 109–10
  Three-Bean Chili, 100–01
  Vegetable and Bean Ragout over
    Couscous, 106–07
  White Bean Stew, 104–05
Stir-Fry, Broccoli-Mushroom, with Tofu,
  125–27
Stir-Fry, Mixed Vegetable, 123–24
stock, vegetable, 88–89
Strawberries, Citrus-Spritzed, 247–48
Strawberry Frozen Dessert, 241–42
stuffed cabbage, 156–57
Stuffed Red Pepper, 148–49
supertasters, cruciferous vegetables and,
  17
Super Toast with Ginger Yogurt,
  69–70
Sutherland, Barbara, 4
Sweet and Sour Bok Choy and Tempeh,
  132–33

Sweet and Sour Chicken, 140–41
Sweet and Sour Tofu, 127–28
Swordfish, Grilled, with Roasted Corn
  and Red Pepper Salsa, 146–47
Swordfish Kebobs, 159

tamari soy sauce, 15
Tangy Tofu Dressing, 201–02
Tapioca, Lychee, 225–26
Tapioca, Mandarin and Bing Cherry,
  231–32
Tapioca Pudding, 242–43
tartar sauce, 151
Tart, Cheese, with Kiwi and Strawber-
  ries, 250–51
tempeh
  about, 13
  recipes using:
  Black Bean and Rice Soup, 101–02
  Linguini with Lentils, 157–58
  Open-Face Lentil-Nut Loaf Sand-
    wich, 111–12
  Spaghetti with Tomato-Tempeh
    Sauce, 151–53
  Sweet and Sour Bok Choy and
    Tempeh, 132–33
  Tempeh with Snow Peas, Mushrooms,
    and Carrots, 49–50
Tempeh with Snow Peas, Mushrooms,
  and Carrots, 49–50
terms
  cooking, 21–22
  other, 23
Thai Soup, 93–94
Three-Bean Chili, 100–01
Toast, Super, with Ginger Yogurt, 69–70
tofu
  about, 13
  recipes using:
  Artichoke Frittata, 74–76
  Broccoli-Mushroom Stir-Fry with
    Tofu, 125–27
  Cauliflower and Carrot Curry with
    Tofu, 131–32
  Curried Tofu, 52–53
  Egg Foo Yung, 58–59
  Enoki Mushroom Custard, 54–55
  Fajitas, 154–55
  Greek Sandwich, 117–18 ·
  Lasagna, 160–61

tofu (*continued*)
  Miso Soup, 53–54
  Mixed Vegetable Stir-Fry, 123–24
  Mu Shu Vegetables, 124–25
  Noodles with Celery, Carrot, and
    Broccoli, 141–42
  Rice Noodles with Vegetables and
    Tofu in Black Bean Sauce, 135–36
  Savory Breakfast Roll, 79–81
  Smoked Tofu Sandwich, 112–13
  Spicy Noodle Salad, 167–68
  Sweet and Sour Tofu, 127–28
  Tangy Tofu Dressing, 201–02
  tartar sauce, 150–51
  Tofu Kebobs, 137–38
  Tofu-Mushroom Soup, 91–92
  Tuna Melt, 114–15
  Vegetables and Tofu with Noodles,
    128–29
Tofu Kebobs, 137–38
Tofu-Mushroom Soup, 91–92
Tomatoes, Baked Roma, with Fresh
  Basil, 198
Tomatoes, Grilled Marinated Mush-
  rooms and, 57–58
Tomatoes, Roma, with Olive Oil, 216
Tomato Salad, Mixed Greens and, 212–
  13
Tricolor Pasta with Tomato and Soybean
  Sauce, 164–65
Trout Fillets, Baked, 163–64
Tuna, Grilled Fresh, 134–35
Tuna-Asparagus Salad, 166–67
Tuna Melt, 114–15

Vegetable and Barley Salad, 176–77
Vegetable and Bean Ragout over Couscous, 106–07
Vegetables and Tofu with Noodles,
  128–29
vegetable dishes. *See also individual
  vegetables*; salads, main-dish; salads,
  side
  Crispy Noodles with Vegetables,
    56–57
  Fresh Soybeans and Vegetables with
    Black Bean Sauce, 130–31

  Fresh Vegetable Medley, 194–95
  Green Cabbage Stuffed with Bulgur
    and Vegetables, 156–57
  Mixed Vegetable Stir-Fry, 123–24
  Mu Shu Vegetables, 124–25
  Ratatouille, 109–10
  Rice and Vegetables, 48
  Rice Noodles with Vegetables and
    Tofu in Black Bean Sauce,
    135–36
  Vegetable and Bean Ragout over
    Couscous, 106–07
  Vegetable and Tofu with Noodles,
    128–29
  Vegetable Pho, 50–51
vegetable gravy, 89
Vegetable Pho, 50–51
Vegetable-Potato Salad, 169–70
vegetables. *See also individual vegeta-
    bles*; vegetable dishes
  containing indole-3–carbinol, 17
  health benefits of, 18–19
vegetable stock, 88–89
Vietnamese Salad Rolls, 208–09
vitamin D, breast cancer and, 18

Waffles, Cornmeal, with Peaches and
  Berries, 76–77
Walnuts with Vanilla Topping, Fresh
  Figs and, 237–38
Water Chestnut Salad, Celery and,
  206–07
Watercress Salad, 204
weight, conversion table, 22
White Bean Stew, 104–05
white sauce, 90
whole grains, about, 18
wild rice, cooking instructions, 179
Wilted Baby Bok Choy, 195–96
wraps
  Breakfast Aram, 86–87
  Rice Wraps, 59–61
  Vietnamese Salad Rolls, 208–09

Yogurt, Ginger, 236–37